ATLAS OF

# VASCULAR SURGERY

*Operative Procedures*

# ATLAS OF
# VASCULAR
# SURGERY

## *Operative Procedures*

**KENNETH OURIEL, M.D.**
Associate Professor of Surgery
Section of Vascular Surgery
University of Rochester
School of Medicine and Dentistry
Rochester, New York


**ROBERT B. RUTHERFORD, M.D.**
Professor of Surgery
University of Colorado Health Sciences Center
Denver, Colorado

*Illustrations by Richard A. Gersony and John Foerster
with assistance from Tom McCracken*

**W.B. SAUNDERS COMPANY**
*A Division of Harcourt Brace & Company*

Philadephia    London    Toronto    Montreal    Sydney    Tokyo

**W.B. SAUNDERS COMPANY**

*A Division of Harcourt Brace & Company*

The Curtis Center
Independence Square West
Philadelphia, Pennsylvania 19106

**Library of Congress Cataloging-in-Publication Data**

Ouriel, Kenneth.
    Atlas of vascular surgery: operative procedures / Kennneth Ouriel, Robert B. Rutherford; illustrations by Richard A. Gersony and John Foerster with assistance from Tom McCracken.

p.    cm.

ISBN 0–7216–6994–8

1.  Blood–vessels—Surgery—Atlases.    I. Rutherford,    Robert    B.    II. Title.
    [DNLM:    1.   Vascular    Surgery—methods—atlases.    WG    17    093a    1998]
    RD598.5.094    1998

617.4′13—dc21

DNLM/DLC                                                                97-22033

ATLAS OF VASCULAR SURGERY: OPERATIVE PROCEDURES               ISBN 0–7216–6994–8

Printed in the United States of America.

Last digit is the print number:      9      8      7      6      5      4      3      2      1

# *PREFACE*___

This atlas of peripheral vascular surgery represents a long-awaited supplement to *Atlas of Vascular Surgery: Basic Techniques and Exposures.* The focus of this book is common peripheral vascular techniques, each of which involves a variety of individual approaches to specific vascular structures as well as strategies designed to most easily accomplish the particular reconstructive procedure.

The contemporary practice of medicine attempts to integrate the myriad scientific disciplines involved in the care of patients; the practice of surgery represents the quintessential example, in which knowledge of anatomy, physiology, and pathology is applied to the treatment of disease processes. The peripheral vascular surgeon in particular must incorporate medical and surgical principles to a greater extent than many subspecialists. Unlike the cardiac surgeon, who works with a cardiologist, and the neurosurgeon, who works with a neurologist, often the vascular surgeon is solely responsible for the clinical diagnosis, treatment, and long-term patient care.

To be complete, an atlas of peripheral vascular surgical operations must include information on clinical diagnosis and perioperative patient care, in addition to a description of the technical maneuvers necessary to perform the particular operative procedure. In this regard, the authors have endeavored to include the information necessary to the formulation of clinical decisions. Operative techniques are presented in detail, emphasizing the clinical setting and the scientific rationale for their undertaking, in hopes of instilling sound judgment in the novice and reinforcing it in the established practitioner.

The techniques in this atlas compose a compendium of operative approaches formulated by applying the knowledge passed to us by our teachers and modified by years of trial and error. Each chapter is related to an individual peripheral vascular operation, and the chapters are grouped into sections according to disease processes. Each chapter begins with a short discussion of clinical pathophysiology, covering treatment indications and options. The operative procedure follows and is discussed in enough detail to provide an understandable commentary for the accompanying illustrations. It is advantageous to keep *Basic Techniques and Exposures* handy when using the present text, because it was not feasible to duplicate all the details of operative exposure here. This approach is  particularly worthwhile for the surgeon in training.

Clearly, a diversity of technical variations exists, in addition to those provided in this text. In fact, the two authors occasionally differ in their individual approaches to given clinical situations. In these instances each operative strategy, with its advantages and its potential drawbacks, is fully described. It is hoped that the procedures included herein will stimulate others to formulate newer operative innovations, just as the authors have been stimulated to improve on the techniques originally learned from their mentors.

KENNETH OURIEL
ROBERT B. RUTHERFORD

# CONTENTS____

## SECTION 3

### *Aneurysm Resection*        *93*

## SECTION 4

### *Renal and Visceral Arterial*
### *Reconstruction*        *143*

# SECTION 5

## *Brachiocephalic Reconstruction*      *189*

# SECTION 6

## *Thoracic Outlet Syndrome*      *249*

# SECTION 7

## *Venous Procedures*      *261*

# INFRAINGUINAL ARTERIAL RECONSTRUCTION

# CHAPTER 1

# Reversed Saphenous Vein Femoropopliteal Bypass

Infrainguinal arterial occlusive disease is one of the most common problems encountered in the practice of vascular surgery. Patients present with symptoms of claudication when the disease is of moderate severity, involving only one arterial segment. The risk of limb loss is low in this group of patients, but failure of an arterial reconstruction performed for claudication may result in thrombosis of arterial segments above or below the procedure, with the development of a nonviable extremity. For this reason, claudication is not considered to be an appropriate indication for arterial reconstruction unless the symptoms truly limit the patient's lifestyle.

Patients with multisegment arterial occlusion frequently manifest pain at rest, ulceration, and gangrene. These findings indicate inadequate arterial perfusion, even at rest, and are harbingers of subsequent limb loss. Whenever possible, patients presenting with these signs and symptoms should be offered revascularization to avoid amputation.

Several options are available for restoring arterial continuity, but the reversed saphenous vein bypass graft is the standard with which all other infrainguinal techniques must be compared. Devised and developed in the late 1940s, reversed vein bypass grafts provide a safe and durable means of bridging across arterial obstructions. The procedure is remarkably independent of the length of the graft or the size of the outflow vessel. The excellent operative results have provided the opportunity to avoid major amputation in patients with marked degrees of ischemia and extensive tissue defects—clinical situations thought unsalvageable even one decade ago.

There exist only three prerequisites for a successful arterial bypass procedure: adequate inflow, suitable outflow, and an appropriate conduit. Preoperative arteriography is essential to plan the sites of inflow and outflow. Preoperative duplex ultrasound vein mapping has gained widespread acceptance in predicting the adequacy of the conduit.

## OPERATIVE PROCEDURE

The operation is begun with exposure of the saphenous vein over the length of planned use. Our preference is to perform autogenous vein bypasses to the below-knee popliteal artery, even in the presence of an apparently adequate above-knee vessel. The proximal popliteal artery is frequently quite diseased, and an above-knee outflow site is chosen only when the length of available vein cannot reach below the knee. In this regard, a very small vein (<3.5 mm in the outer dimension) or a vein that has been the site of previous superficial phlebitis would be deemed unusable. The surgeon should not persist in the harvest of a clearly inadequate vein; the results of prosthetic bypass are superior to those associated with the use of an inadequate venous conduit, regardless of the site of outflow.

The saphenous vein is excised from the mid-calf to the groin, ligating tributaries with 3-0 silk suture. The harvest incision is placed directly over the vein to avoid development of flap necrosis. The inflow and outflow arteries can be exposed through the vein harvest incision *without* the formation of a tenuous skin flap, because these structures lie much deeper than the vein.

Several caveats of vein harvest are worthy of mention (Fig. 1). First, the vein should be kept moist during harvest (Fig. 2). The lights of the operating theater tend to

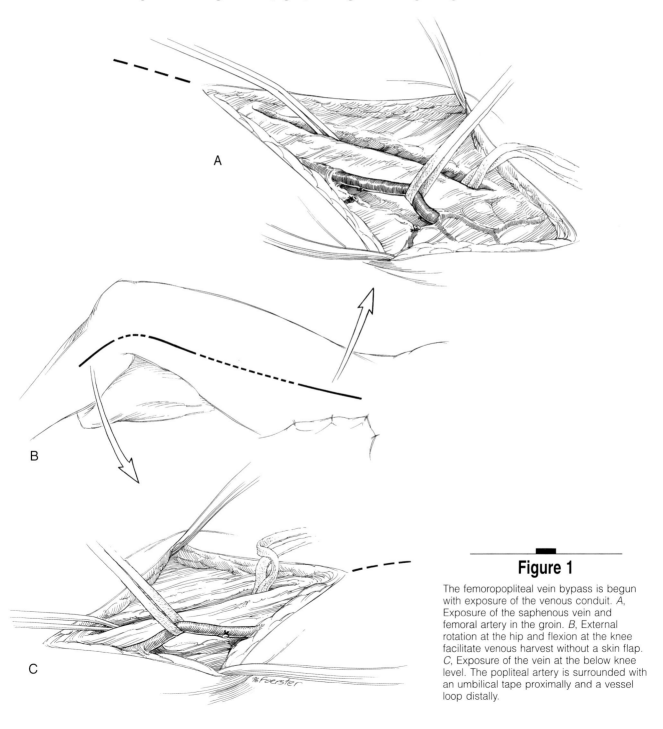

## Figure 1

The femoropopliteal vein bypass is begun with exposure of the venous conduit. *A,* Exposure of the saphenous vein and femoral artery in the groin. *B,* External rotation at the hip and flexion at the knee facilitate venous harvest without a skin flap. *C,* Exposure of the vein at the below knee level. The popliteal artery is surrounded with an umbilical tape proximally and a vessel loop distally.

## *Reversed Saphenous Vein Femoropopliteal Bypass*

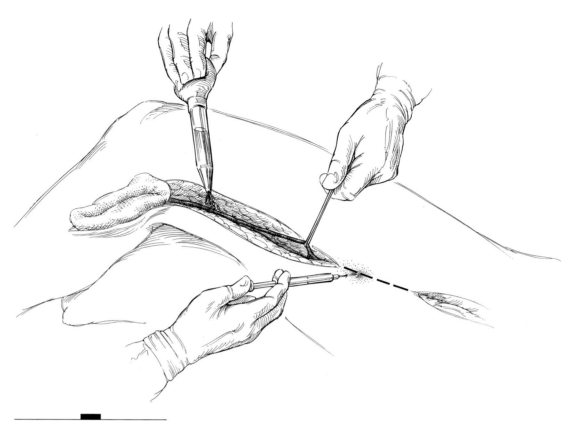

## Figure 2

Harvest of the greater saphenous vein, using various techniques to minimize trauma to the conduit. The exposed vein is kept from desiccation by using moist packs and saline irrigation. Vessel loops are used to hold the vein. The subcutaneous tissue overlying the vein may be infiltrated with papaverine or lidocaine to prevent spasm.

dry the vein. Second, grasping it with forceps can injure the vein. We have found a Silastic loop useful in retraction, but only the adventitia of the vein should be grasped if DeBakey forceps are employed. Third, some surgeons prefer the use of subcutaneous heparin and papaverine injection to prevent spasm of the vein. We have not employed this technique for reversed vein bypasses; we instead gently dilate the vein with a heparinized papaverine solution after excision. Open tributaries that were missed during harvest are grasped with fine forceps and ligated with silk suture at this time (Fig. 3).

After harvest, the vein is reversed. Placement of the vein beneath the muscular layers may be beneficial if the wound is thought to be tenuous. In this case, the vein is tunneled between the heads of the gastrocnemius muscle (Fig. 4) or beneath the sartorius

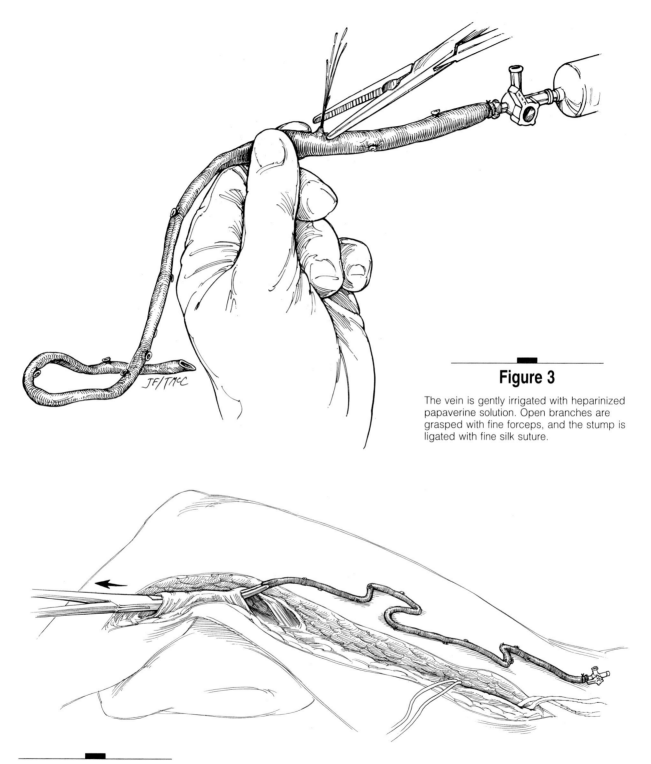

**Figure 3**

The vein is gently irrigated with heparinized papaverine solution. Open branches are grasped with fine forceps, and the stump is ligated with fine silk suture.

**Figure 4**

The vein is tunneled subfascially between the heads of the gastrocnemius muscle to reach the infragenicular popliteal artery. This approach prevents exposure of the graft in case wound problems develop.

## *Reversed Saphenous Vein Femoropopliteal Bypass*

muscle (Fig. 5) to prevent exposure of the graft if the wound separates. The patient is administered heparin, and the proximal anastomosis is constructed with 6-0 running polypropylene suture (Fig. 6). The distal anastomosis is completed in a similar fashion (Fig. 7). Flow is restored, and hemostasis is secured, with or without protamine reversal of the heparin effect.

Intraoperative interrogation of the graft using duplex scanning or arteriography is wise. Simple Doppler evaluation may not be sensitive enough to detect vein graft stenotic lesions or anastomotic defects. After the adequacy of the hemodynamic result has been established, the wounds are closed with running subcutaneous absorbable suture and clips or running subcuticular suture for the skin.

The long-term patency of vein grafts may be improved through the use of postoperative surveillance with duplex ultrasonography. The graft should be thoroughly examined before discharge from the hospital and at the time of the first postoperative outpatient visit. Duplex scans are repeated every 3 months for 2 years and then regularly but less frequently thereafter.

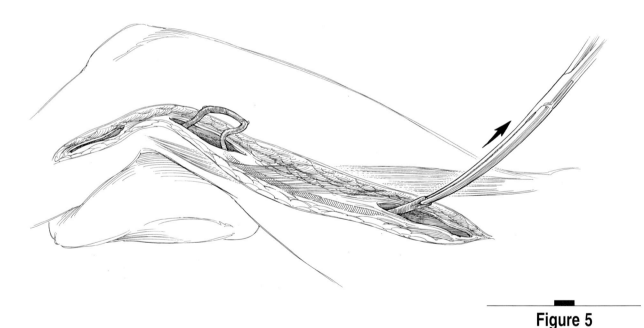

## Figure 5

The vein is tunneled subsartorially when the risk of postoperative wound problems is great.

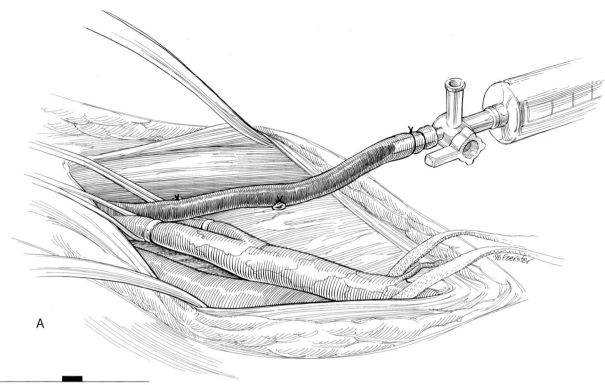

A

## Figure 6

*A*, The femoral bifurcation is exposed in the
groin. *B*, Proximal anastomosis is complete.

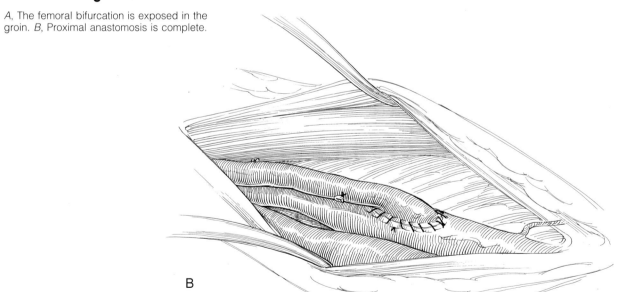

B

*Reversed Saphenous Vein Femoropopliteal Bypass*

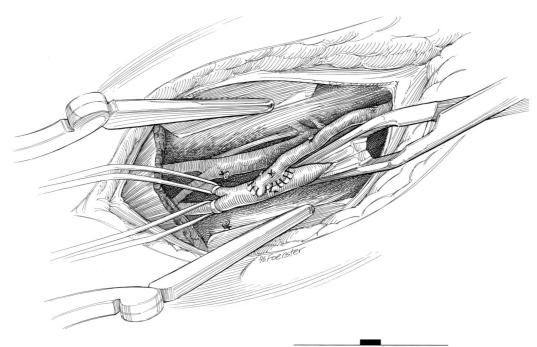

**Figure 7**

The distal anastomosis on the infragenicular popliteal artery is complete.

# CHAPTER 2

# Femoral to Above-Knee Popliteal Bypass With ePTFE

Prosthetic conduits represent acceptable alternatives to an autogenous graft when the above-knee popliteal artery is suitable for outflow. Some authorities have recommended the preferential use of a prosthetic graft when the distal anastomosis can be kept above the level of the knee joint. We prefer to employ greater saphenous vein when available, but logical arguments can be made to the contrary. First, the patency rate of Dacron and ePTFE conduits has been demonstrated to be substantially equivalent to that associated with vein grafts when the distal anastomosis is above the knee. Second, the use of a prosthetic graft allows the preservation of vein for a subsequent, more distal bypass procedure or for coronary artery bypass. Third, a prosthetic femoral popliteal reconstruction requires two relatively short incisions, reducing the period of recovery.

## OPERATIVE PROCEDURE

The patient is placed in the supine position with the hip externally rotated and the knee partly flexed. The leg, groin, and lower abdomen are sterilely prepared and draped (Fig. 8). A longitudinal groin incision is made over the common femoral artery. It is important to note that the inguinal ligament may actually lie well superior to the groin crease in patients with a large abdominal pannus. Prior palpation for the pubic tubercle and anterior superior iliac spine will avoid the error of placing the groin incision too low. The incision is usually placed with at least one third of its length above the inguinal crease. The complete incision may be placed above the inguinal crease in obese individuals, and a transverse configuration can avoid the crease and may decrease the risk of postoperative wound infection. The subcutaneous tissues are divided, ligating any lymphatic channels that are encountered. The lower border of the inguinal ligament is identified, and the common femoral artery is unroofed. The vessel is followed to its bifurcation into the superficial femoral and profunda femoris arteries, and each branch is surrounded with a vessel loop (Fig. 9).

## *Femoral to Above-Knee Popliteal Bypass With ePTFE*

Distal exposure is facilitated by external rotation at the hip and flexion at the knee, with the placement of a bolster beneath the calf. The inappropriate placement of a bolster above the level of the knee pushes the posterior thigh muscles medially, obstructing the operator's view of the popliteal vessels. An incision is made in the crease palpated between the sartorius and vastus medialis muscles, running from the medial femoral condyle to a point overlying the adductor magnus tendon (Fig. 10). The sartorius muscle is retracted posteriorly, and the loose fascia overlying the popliteal space is divided. A large popliteal vein is readily encountered, and retracting the vein in a posteromedial direction exposes the popliteal artery. The artery is palpated for disease, choosing a segment suitable for anastomosis. When more distal exposure of the popliteal artery is required, partial division of the medial head of the gastrocnemius muscle allows additional exposure of the suprageenicular vessel. If the occlusive process reaches the level of the mid-knee, as revealed on an anteroposterior arteriographic view, suprageenicular bypass is not feasible.

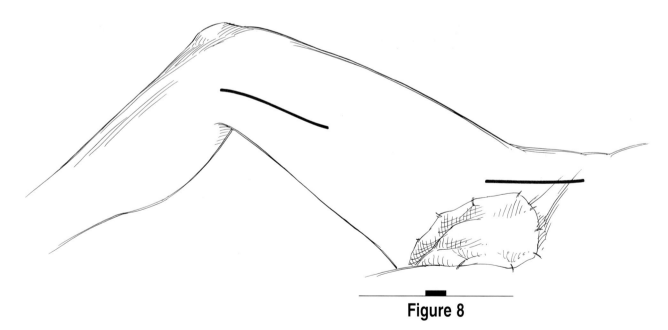

## Figure 8

The patient's leg is externally rotated for placement of a femoral to above-knee popliteal prosthetic graft. The femoral incision is placed at the level of the inguinal ligament, and the popliteal incision runs from the medial condyle of the femur to a point overlying the adductor hiatus.

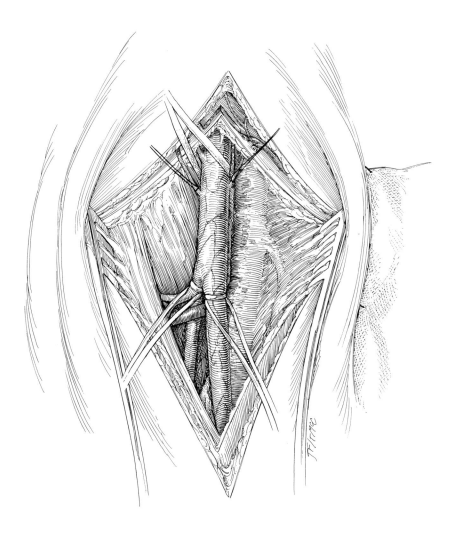

**Figure 9**

The common femoral, superficial femoral, and profunda femoris arteries are exposed in the groin.

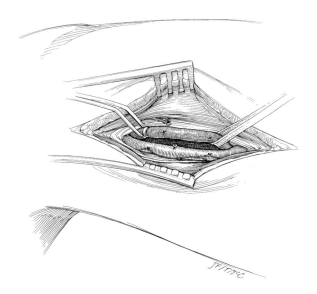

**Figure 10**

The above-knee popliteal artery is exposed in the groove between the sartorius and vastus medialis muscles.

## *Femoral to Above-Knee Popliteal Bypass With ePTFE*

Before heparinization, the graft (6 or 8 mm in diameter) is tunneled beneath the sartorius muscle but superficial to the adductor magnus tendon (Fig. 11). It is easiest to pass the tunneling instrument from the lower thigh incision to the groin incision, fighting to keep the tip of the tunneler as superficial as possible during advancement. Otherwise, the instrument tends to track deep below the muscular floor of the femoral triangle, below the femoral artery.

The patient is administered heparin, and the graft is sewn in place, preferentially performing the proximal and distal anastomoses simultaneously with a two-team approach. As with all infrainguinal bypasses, the graft length is determined with the knee extended; otherwise, the conduit will be too short. The graft is beveled (Fig. 12), and the popliteal anastomosis is completed in an end-to-side fashion (Fig. 13). We use Gore-Tex suture (6-0 or 7-0) with ePTFE grafts because of decreased suture-hole bleeding.

When an extraordinarily diseased popliteal artery is encountered, it may be difficult of locate the vessel lumen with a simple longitudinal arteriotomy. An end-to-end distal anastomosis should be considered in these instances, because it provides circumferential tacking of the dense plaque and avoids inadvertent anastomosis to a false channel of the artery.

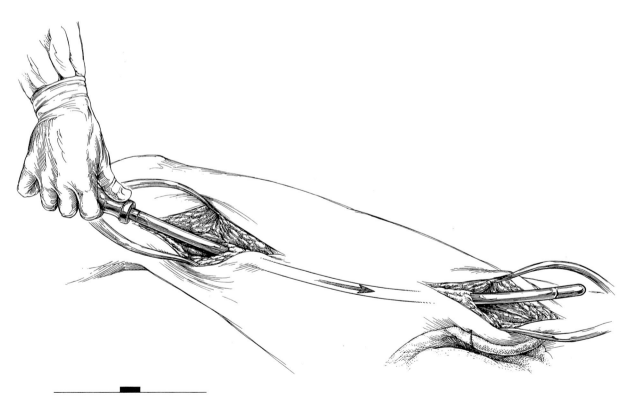

## Figure 11

The graft is placed beneath the sartorius muscle with the aid of a metallic tunneling device.

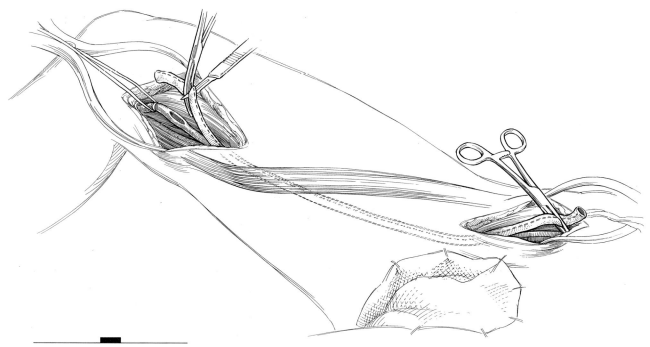

## Figure 12

The graft is beveled for the anastomoses using a curved hemostat and the knife blade.

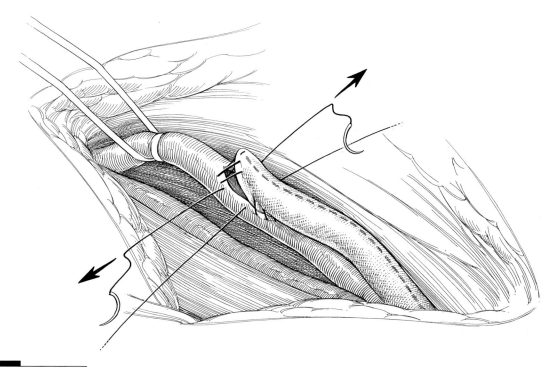

## Figure 13

Completion of the popliteal anastomosis is achieved using a two-suture technique.

## Femoral to Above-Knee Popliteal Bypass With ePTFE

The femoral anastomosis is most easily performed without the external hip rotation used for the distal exposure (Fig. 14). The femoral anastomosis is completed with running Gore-Tex suture (Fig. 15), and the clamps are released. An adequate technical result is checked with digital palpation of the pulse just beyond the anastomosis (Fig. 16), Doppler assessment of distal pulses, or duplex ultrasound. Intraoperative arteriography should be performed in difficult cases with the injection of contrast (usually 20 ml) through the graft (Fig. 17). Inadequate images may be result if the inflow and profunda vessels are not clamped during dye injection.

Protamine sulfate is administered at the discretion of the surgeon but is unnecessary in many cases. After securing hemostasis, the wounds are closed with running absorbable suture for the subcutaneous layer and clips or subcuticular suture for the skin. Postoperatively, the ankle-brachial index is recorded and followed on a regular basis after discharge.

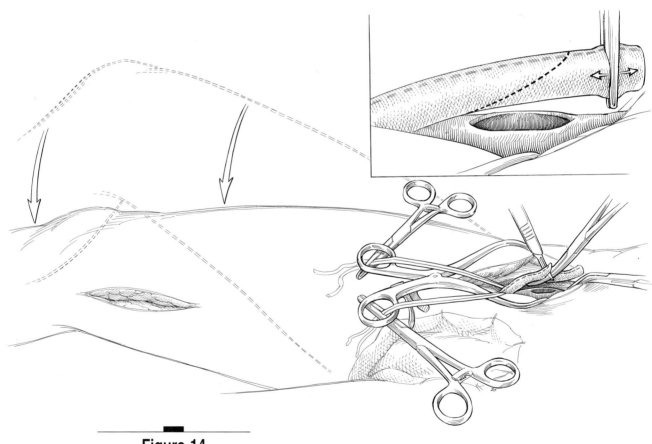

### Figure 14

Completion of the proximal anastomosis. It is advantageous, although not mandatory, to release the external leg rotation during performance of the femoral anastomosis. The graft is cut, taking care to match the length of the beveled graft to the length of the arteriotomy (inset).

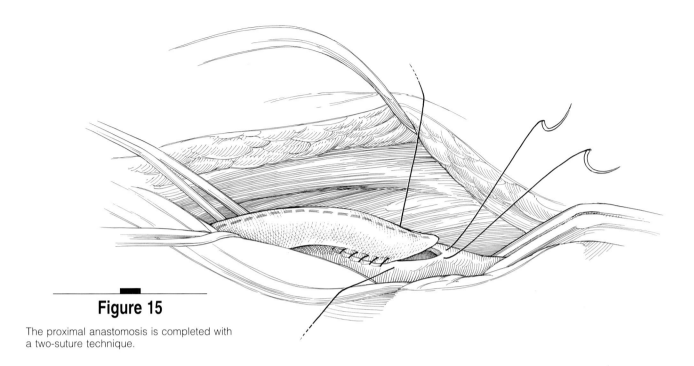

## Figure 15

The proximal anastomosis is completed with a two-suture technique.

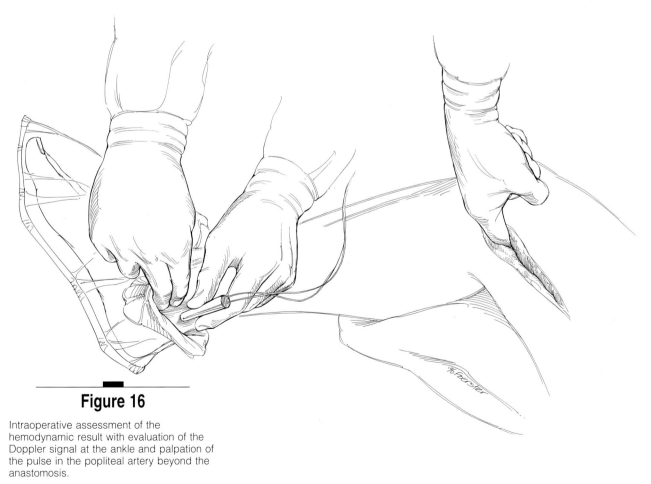

## Figure 16

Intraoperative assessment of the hemodynamic result with evaluation of the Doppler signal at the ankle and palpation of the pulse in the popliteal artery beyond the anastomosis.

## *Femoral to Above-Knee Popliteal Bypass With ePTFE*

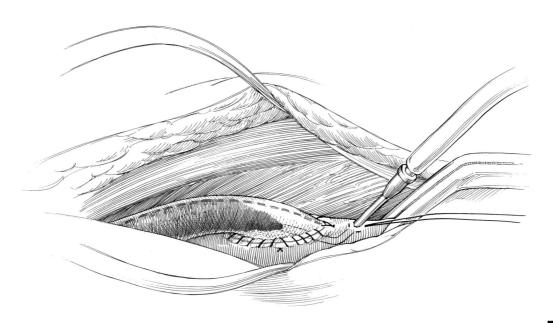

**Figure 17**

Intraoperative arteriography is performed by placing a right-angled cannula through the femoral artery just proximal to the anastomosis. A U-stitch is in place to arrest bleeding after removal of the cannula.

# CHAPTER 3

# In Situ Saphenous Vein Femoropopliteal Bypass

The in situ bypass technique, originally conceived by Drs. Rob and Hall in 1959, was reintroduced and popularized 20 years thereafter by Drs. Leather and Karmody. An in situ bypass differs from a reversed vein bypass with respect to the direction of the vein in relation to blood flow. In the in situ technique, the vein is left in its original bed, and the venous valves are rendered incompetent. Herein lies the major risk of the in situ technique—the process of destroying the venous valves may injure the fragile venous endothelium. Occasionally, the valve-cutting instrument may catch a branch orifice and lacerate the vein wall, and a patch angioplasty or excision and reanastomosis is then required. A second problem is created by the failure to ligate venous tributaries, which for large tributaries can result in troublesome postoperative arteriovenous fistulae and a steal of nutrient blood flow from the leg.

The theoretical advantages of the in situ technique are several. First, the large end of the vein is placed on the larger inflow artery, and the smaller end of the vein is placed on the smaller, outflow vessel (Fig. 18). This advantage may seem less important when performing a bypass to the most distal vessels, because the saphenous vein at the malleolar level is usually relatively large in caliber. Second, leaving the vein in its bed may allow continued nourishment of the venous wall through preserved vasa vasorum. Third, the venous valves in a reversed vein graft may function as mild stenoses, the hemodynamic significance of which is correlated with the flow through the graft and the number of valves in series. Although the valves have few hemodynamic effects at the level of flow observed in the venous circulation, the greater flows observed when arterialized may produce a pressure drop across the graft. These hemodynamic aberrations may be ameliorated when the valves are disrupted, because the normal, open venous valve has a greater resistance to flow than the nonreversed, disrupted valve.

## *In Situ Saphenous Vein Femoropopliteal Bypass*

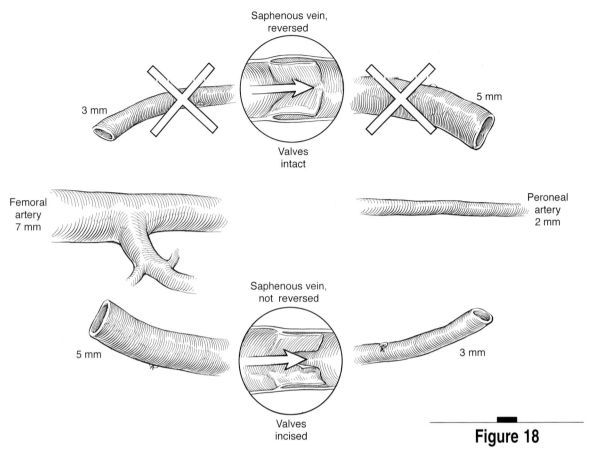

**Figure 18**

The advantages of in situ saphenous vein bypass include the ability to place the large end of the vein on the large artery and the small end of the vein on the smaller artery. Flow through the lysed valve leaflets may be greater than flow through nonlysed, reversed leaflets.

# OPERATIVE PROCEDURE

An in situ bypass may be performed without exposing the vein along its complete length (Fig. 19). Until the operator is thoroughly familiar with the in situ technique, however, complete exposure is safest. The vein is unroofed throughout its course, with visualization and ligation of the tributaries. The outflow vessel is exposed, mobilizing a suitable length of corresponding saphenous vein. In the case of posterior tibial outflow, only a short length of vein must be mobilized. A somewhat longer segment of vein should be mobilized to reach to the below-knee popliteal or the peroneal artery. Bypass to the anterior tibial artery requires mobilization of a rather long venous segment to bridge the gap around the tibia or through the interosseous membrane.

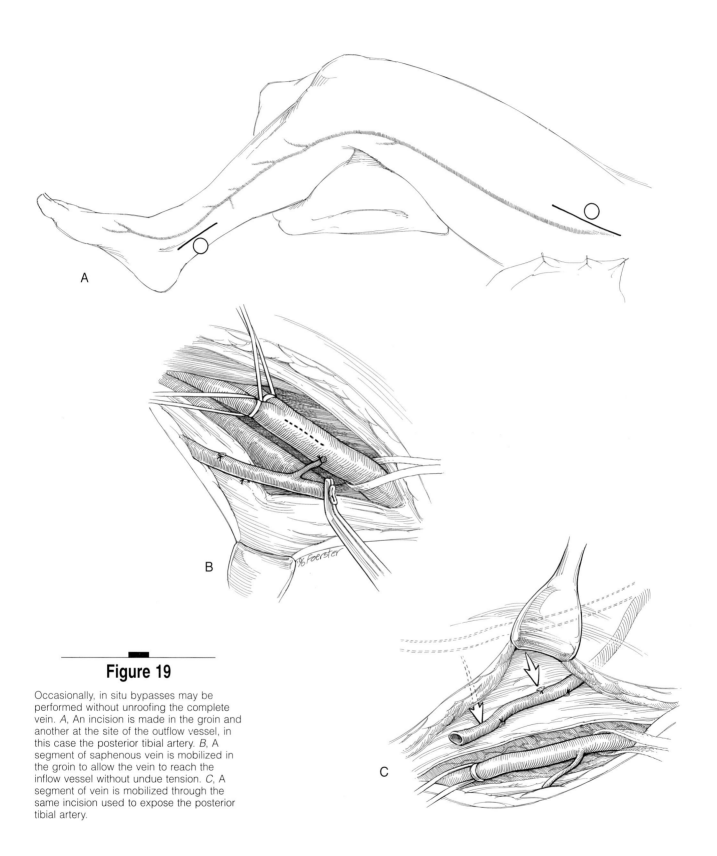

## Figure 19

Occasionally, in situ bypasses may be
performed without unroofing the complete
vein. *A*, An incision is made in the groin and
another at the site of the outflow vessel, in
this case the posterior tibial artery. *B*, A
segment of saphenous vein is mobilized in
the groin to allow the vein to reach the
inflow vessel without undue tension. *C*, A
segment of vein is mobilized through the
same incision used to expose the posterior
tibial artery.

### *In Situ Saphenous Vein Femoropopliteal Bypass*

Large tributaries should be preserved for introduction of a Mills valvulotome, probably the most precise of the valvulotomy instruments. Complete mobilization of the vein from its bed (the nonreversed bypass technique, Fig. 20) allows safer valve disruption, straightening the vein to minimize the risk of trauma from the valvulotome. Problems associated with the disparity between the termination of the saphenous vein and the common femoral arteriotomy are avoided, because the completely mobilized vein is merely moved to a more proximal location. The nonreversed technique allows the vein graft to be placed in a deep submuscular tunnel in case wound healing problems are anticipated. The same basic technique allows the vein to be transposed to another location and used antegrade to avoid diameter mismatch.

The process of valve disruption begins in the groin, excising the first or first and second valves under direct vision or incising them with a Leather scissors (Fig. 21). A valvulotome of the surgeon's choice is passed from the ankle to the groin; the Leather valve cutter is illustrated in Figure 22. Heparin and papaverine solution is infused into the upper portion of the vein to dilate it and coapt the valves in preparation for cutting. The valve cutter is withdrawn to the level of the knee, but no farther, because the infragenicular saphenous vein may be easily injured with the Leather instrument. At this point, the Leather instrument is removed, and a Mills valvulotome is inserted through the cut end of the vein or through one or more side branches. The Mills instrument is withdrawn, disrupting the valve leaflets in a sequential fashion. An angioscope may be employed to guide the process and prevent inadvertent entrance into a side branch (Fig. 23). A gush of fluid spurts from the distal end after the last valve has been successfully lysed (Fig. 24).

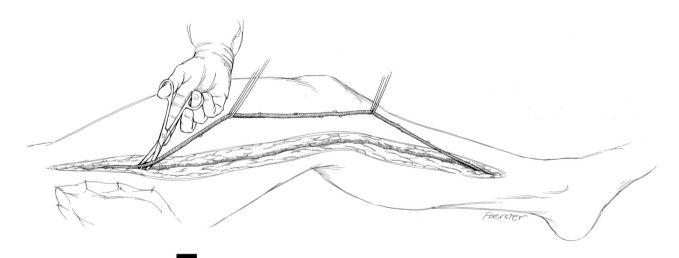

### Figure 20

The vein may be used in a "nonreversed" fashion, mobilizing it entirely from its bed and lysing the valves but maintaining the natural orientation. This method is safest from the standpoint of valve disruption, because it can be done without injury and complete ligation of fistulae. Of necessity, the venous vasa vasorum are disrupted, eliminating a source of nourishment for the venous wall. In theory, the venous endothelium may be less well preserved after complete mobilization.

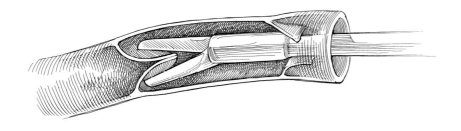

## Figure 21

The first or first and second venous valves are lysed with the Leather scissors. These leaflets may be extremely tough and very difficult to cut with intraluminal valvulotomes and are therefore best addressed under direct or semidirect vision.

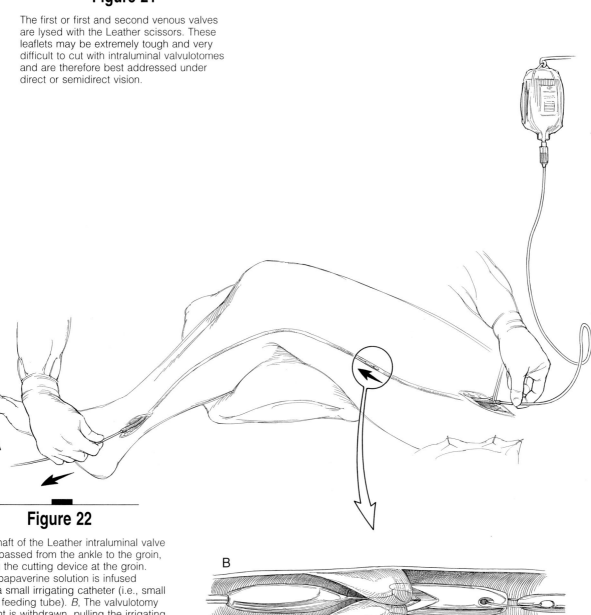

## Figure 22

A, The shaft of the Leather intraluminal valve cutter is passed from the ankle to the groin, attaching the cutting device at the groin. Heparin-papaverine solution is infused through a small irrigating catheter (i.e., small pediatric feeding tube). B, The valvulotomy instrument is withdrawn, pulling the irrigating catheter behind it. The Leather cutter is used only for the larger portion of the vein in the thigh. The lower valves are incised with the Mills valvulotome.

### In Situ Saphenous Vein Femoropopliteal Bypass

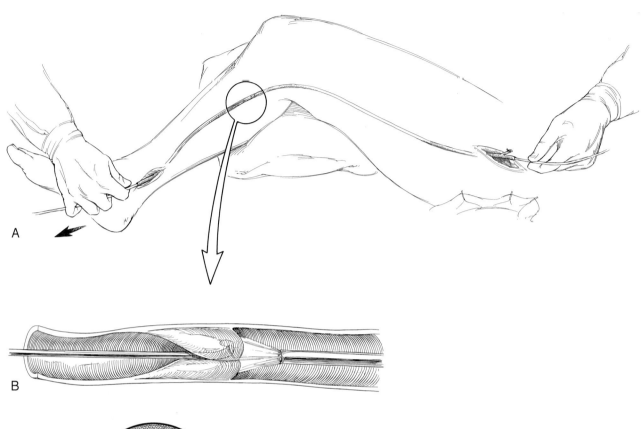

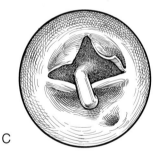

**Figure 23**

*A*, The Mills valvulotome may be used to disrupt the valves of the calf, and an angioscope provides a margin of safety. *B*, The valves are lysed while the surgeon observes the process through the scope. *C*, Angioscopic valve disruption allows the surgeon to avoid inadvertent entry of the valvulotome into a side branch.

The femoral anastomosis is performed after the valves have been disrupted (Fig. 25). If the valves are to be lysed under the pressure of pulsatile blood, however, the proximal anastomosis is performed after cutting only the first or first and second valves. Because the femoral bifurcation and the terminus of the saphenous vein are usually at an identical level, anastomosis to the midportion of the common femoral artery may require mobilization of the vein with or without excision of a tongue of common femoral vein. Alternatively, it may be more efficient to place the proximal anastomosis on the profunda femoris or superficial femoral arteries if they have no proximal stenotic disease. In either case, preservation of a large venous branch provides access for intraoperative arteriography.

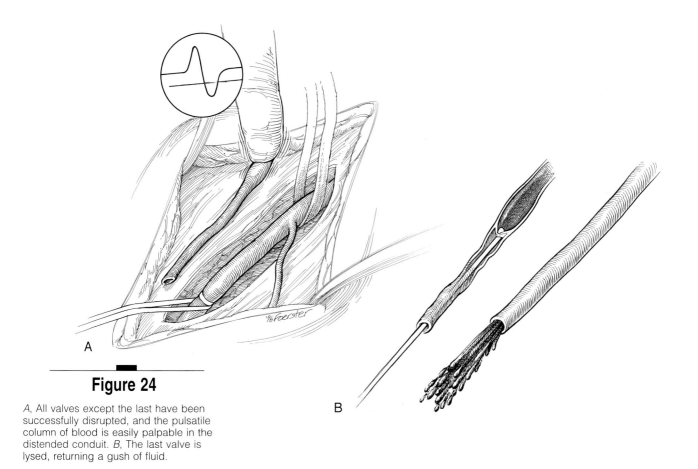

A

B

## Figure 24

*A*, All valves except the last have been successfully disrupted, and the pulsatile column of blood is easily palpable in the distended conduit. *B*, The last valve is lysed, returning a gush of fluid.

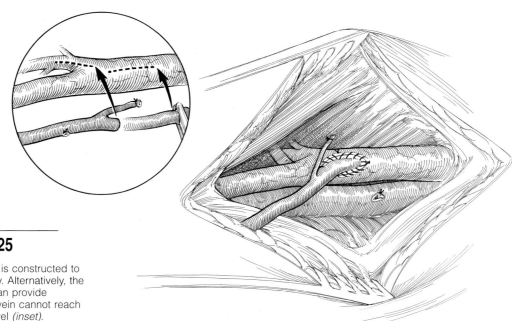

## Figure 25

The proximal anastomosis is constructed to the common femoral artery. Alternatively, the profunda femoris vessel can provide excellent inflow when the vein cannot reach to the common femoral level *(inset)*.

## *In Situ Saphenous Vein Femoropopliteal Bypass*

The distal anastomosis is performed using 6-0 polypropylene suture for popliteal outflow or 7-0 polypropylene suture for infrapopliteal outflow. Infrapopliteal anastomoses are routinely performed using a tourniquet for control, minimizing the extent of tibial artery exposure and decreasing the risk of clamp injury to the small vessels. The posterior tibial artery is exposed through the vein harvest incision, immediately posterior to the saphenous vein at the ankle (Fig. 26). The distal anterior tibial artery requires a second incision for exposure (Fig. 27). The vein is carefully tunneled to the anterior tibial incision (Figs. 28 and 29), and the anastomosis is completed under tourniquet control (Fig. 30).

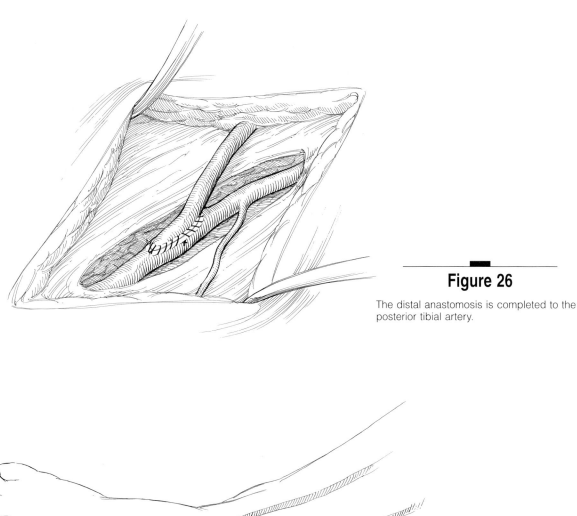

**Figure 26**

The distal anastomosis is completed to the posterior tibial artery.

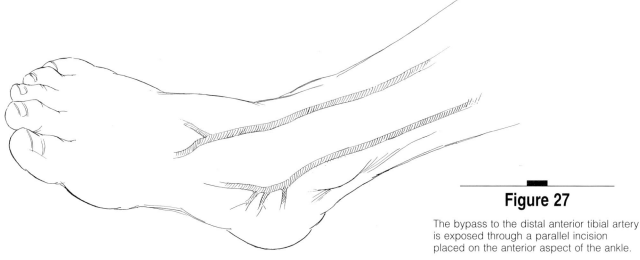

**Figure 27**

The bypass to the distal anterior tibial artery is exposed through a parallel incision placed on the anterior aspect of the ankle.

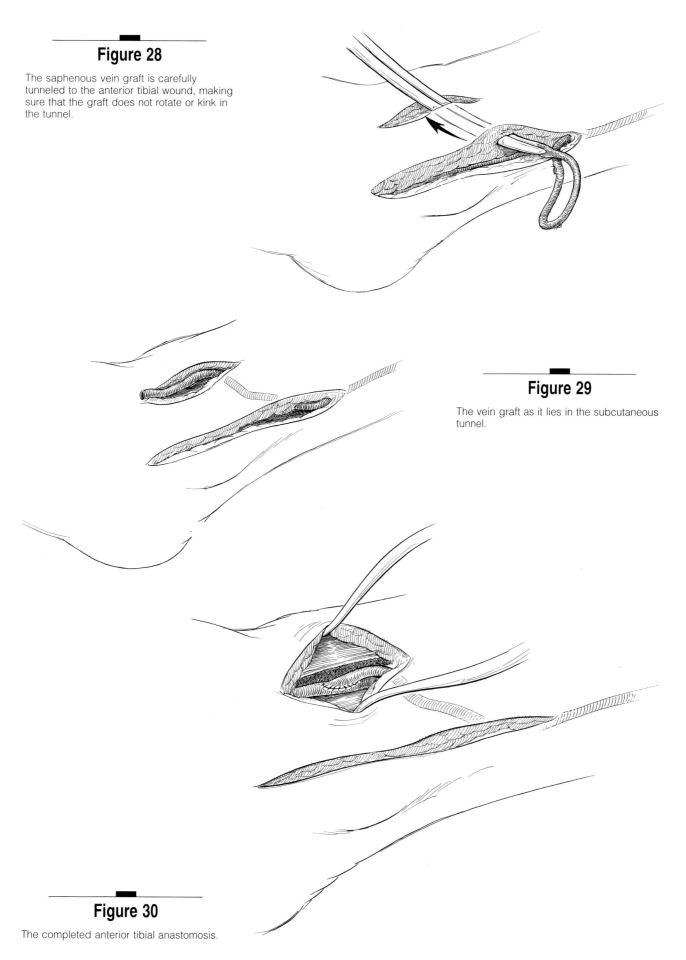

## Figure 28

The saphenous vein graft is carefully tunneled to the anterior tibial wound, making sure that the graft does not rotate or kink in the tunnel.

## Figure 29

The vein graft as it lies in the subcutaneous tunnel.

## Figure 30

The completed anterior tibial anastomosis.

### In Situ Saphenous Vein Femoropopliteal Bypass

The process of identifying the arteriovenous fistulae commences after the anastomoses have been completed. Flow through the vein graft is ascertained with the Doppler instrument positioned just beyond the proximal anastomosis (Fig. 31). Digital occluding pressure is sequentially applied while looking for a large amount of diastolic flow (indicative of an arteriovenous fistula) or an obstructed signal (no fistula). When the location of a fistula has been identified, a small incision is made, and the branch is clipped (Fig. 32). Completion arteriography is performed through a large preserved tributary, with the inflow clamped to improve the image (Fig. 33).

The incisions are closed using absorbable subcutaneous suture for the vein harvest incision and the groin incision and clips or running subcuticular suture for the skin. The incision on the dorsum of the foot is notorious for poor healing. For this reason, extreme care is taken during closure, employing fine nylon interrupted vertical mattress sutures that are loosely tied.

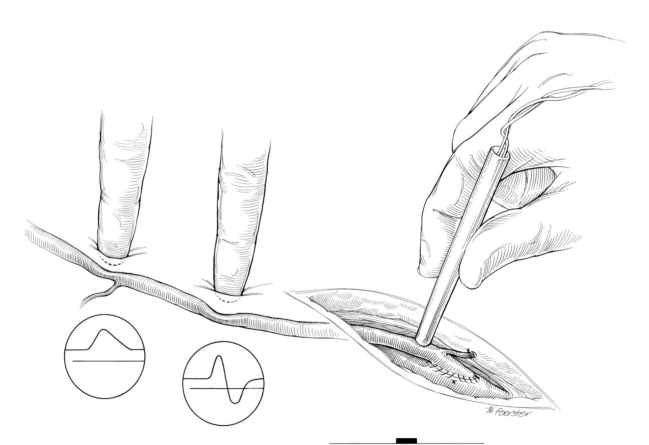

**Figure 31**

Doppler interrogation of an unexposed vein graft to locate arteriovenous fistulae. Digital pressure is applied to the vein graft, beginning just below the groin with serial application of pressure along the length of the graft. An abrupt change in the Doppler signal with increased diastolic flow signifies the presence of a fistula.

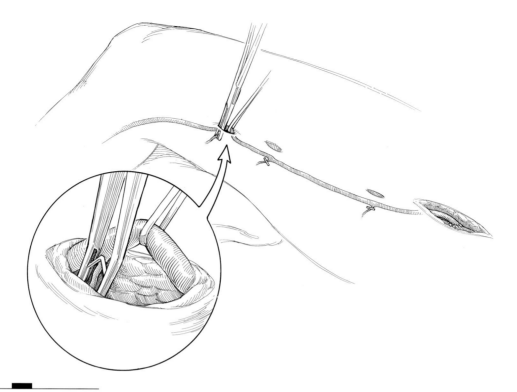

**Figure 32**

Small incisions are placed over the site of each fistula, and the branch is ligated with a hemoclip.

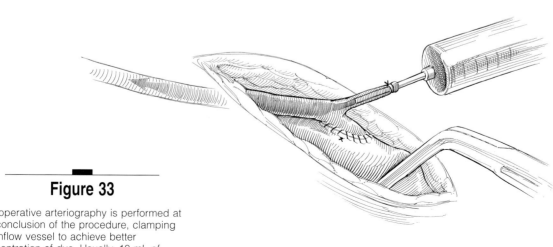

**Figure 33**

Intraoperative arteriography is performed at the conclusion of the procedure, clamping the inflow vessel to achieve better concentration of dye. Usually, 10 mL of contrast provides adequate visualization of the fistulae.

# CHAPTER 4

# Saphenous Vein Popliteal to Dorsalis Pedis Bypass

Infrapopliteal occlusive disease, common in diabetics, frequently results in limb-threatening ischemia with symptoms of pain at rest, ulceration, and gangrene. The pattern is usually one of distal popliteal and proximal tibial artery stenotic lesions; the superficial femoral and proximal popliteal arteries may be remarkably free of disease.

The distal posterior tibial artery is our first choice for outflow in these patients, because the artery communicates directly with the pedal arch, and all but distal-most portion of the artery can be exposed through the same incision used for vein harvest. Anterior tibial outflow, exposed through a lateral lower leg incision, provides pulsatile flow to the foot and is our second choice for outflow in patients with tissue loss in the forefoot. The peroneal artery, however, does not communicate directly with the forefoot and may be associated with a lower chance of healing necrotic wounds of the foot. We reserve the use of the peroneal artery for patients without forefoot tissue loss or in whom the other tibial arteries are occluded.

The arteries of the foot may provide adequate outflow when the crural arteries are occluded. The branches of the posterior tibial artery, the lateral and medial plantar vessels, are ideal outflow sites in this setting. The lateral plantar branch provides somewhat better outflow than the medial branch, because it communicates directly with the plantar arch. The vessels are exposed through an incision placed posterior to the most distal portion of the malleolus, following the distal posterior tibial artery to its bifurcation. The two branches may be differentiated by the somewhat more inferior location of the lateral plantar artery as it begins its lateral course to the plantar arch.

The dorsalis pedis artery is another suitable outflow site when pulsatile forefoot blood flow is required. The artery may be the best distal site in diabetic patients. However, the wound on the dorsum of the foot may be associated with slow healing and separation, resulting in exposure of the bypass graft. These problems have been lessened by avoiding the use of parallel incisions and by ending the vein harvest incision well above the malleoli.

## OPERATIVE PROCEDURE

The patient's entire leg and foot are prepared sterilely. A sterile glove is placed over the forefoot, because it is difficult to adequately prepare the toes or forefoot ulcerations. The greater saphenous vein is harvested from the lower thigh to a point above the medial malleolus (Fig. 34). Parallel incisions are avoided in this manner, decreasing tension during closure of the forefoot wound. Venous side branches are ligated with fine silk, and the vein is prepared for use as a reversed conduit (Fig. 35).

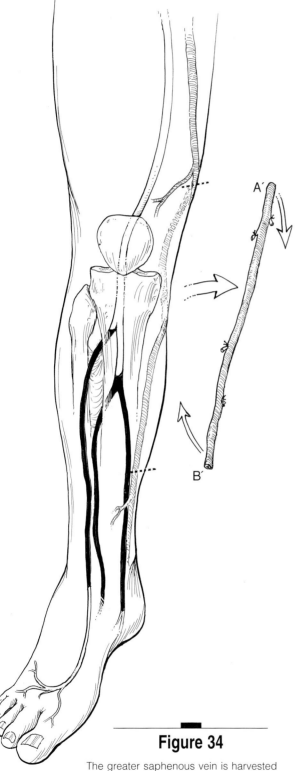

**Figure 34**

The greater saphenous vein is harvested from a supramalleolar level to the lower thigh. The vein is ligated just below a large tributary to preserve flow through the remaining segment and to prevent superficial phlebitis.

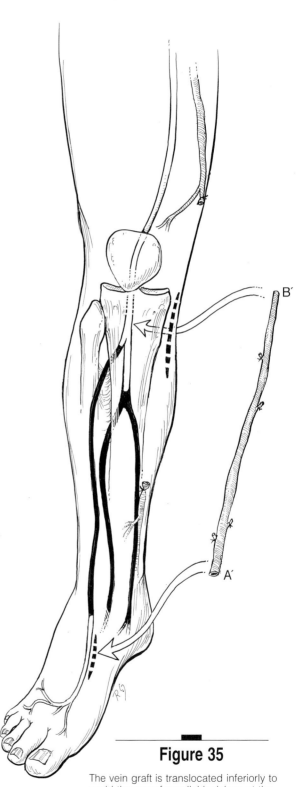

**Figure 35**

The vein graft is translocated inferiorly to avoid the use of parallel incisions at the ankle.

## *Saphenous Vein Popliteal to Dorsalis Pedis Bypass*

The infragenicular popliteal artery is exposed through a medial approach (Fig. 36). The crural fascia is incised, cutting the semimembranosus and semitendinosus tendons when additional proximal exposure is required. Alternatively, the upper portion of the incision can be curved posteriorly to avoid the need to divide the tendons. The popliteal artery is found behind the large popliteal vein and is exposed for a distance of several centimeters (Fig. 37). The proximal anastomosis is completed with 6-0 polypropylene suture (Fig. 38), tunneling the vein in the subcutaneous space to reach the other incision on the dorsum of the foot. It is reasonable to place the vein in a *subfascial* tunnel when the outflow is to a vessel other than the dorsalis pedis artery (e.g., the posterior tibial artery), thereby decreasing the chance of vein graft exposure if wound problems develop.

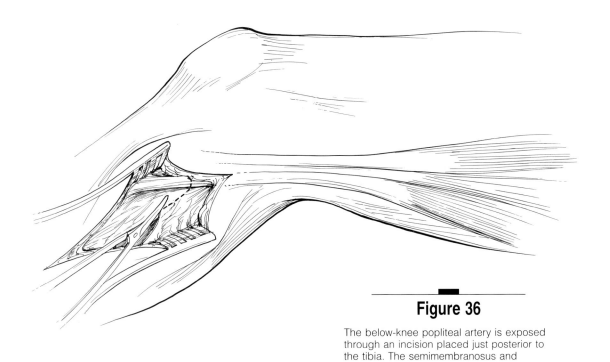

### Figure 36

The below-knee popliteal artery is exposed through an incision placed just posterior to the tibia. The semimembranosus and semitendinosus tendons are severed to obtain additional exposure.

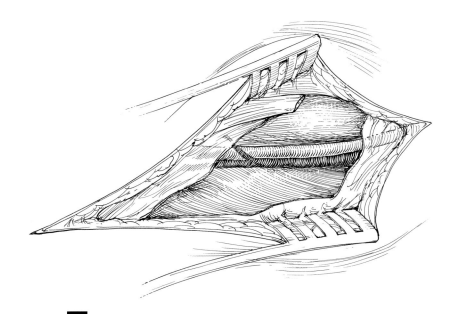

**Figure 37**

The popliteal artery is found deep to the large popliteal vein and is exposed after the vein has been mobilized medially.

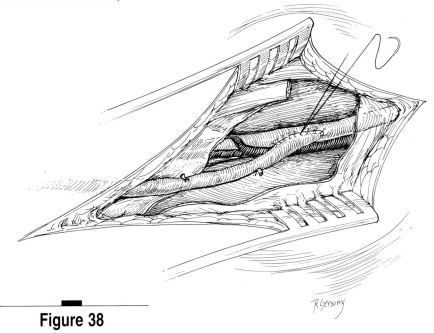

**Figure 38**

The proximal anastomosis is constructed in an end-to-side fashion using 6-0 polypropylene suture.

## Saphenous Vein Popliteal to Dorsalis Pedis Bypass

The dorsalis pedis artery is exposed through a longitudinal incision placed just beyond the skin crease of the ankle (Fig. 39). The dense tissue of the extensor retinaculum is incised, and the artery is found between the extensor hallucis longus and extensor digitorum brevis muscle tendons. A few patients have the dorsalis pedis artery located more laterally than normal. The preoperative identification of the precise location of the vessel can avoid large skin flaps when the incision is inappropriately placed.

The vein is tunneled to the distal incision, taking care to prevent twisting of the conduit in the subcutaneous space. Flow is checked with brief release of the clamp. An occluding tourniquet is placed just above the distal incision and is inflated to suprasystolic pressure after application of an Esmarch bandage. The distal anastomosis is performed with 7-0 polypropylene suture (Fig. 40). The reconstruction is assessed with Doppler, duplex ultrasound, or arteriography after release of the tourniquet. Hemostasis is achieved, and the proximal wound is closed in layers. We routinely close the foot incision with interrupted 4-0 nylon vertical mattress sutures and cover the wound with an occlusive, impervious dressing.

The postoperative patency of the bypass to the foot vessels is roughly equivalent to that of other outflow sites, as long as the saphenous venous conduit is adequate. Patients are treated with antiplatelet agents, and graft surveillance with duplex ultrasound is performed on a quarterly basis for the first 2 years postoperatively.

## Figure 39

The dorsalis pedis artery is exposed on the dorsum of the foot, beneath the dense fascia of the extensor retinaculum.

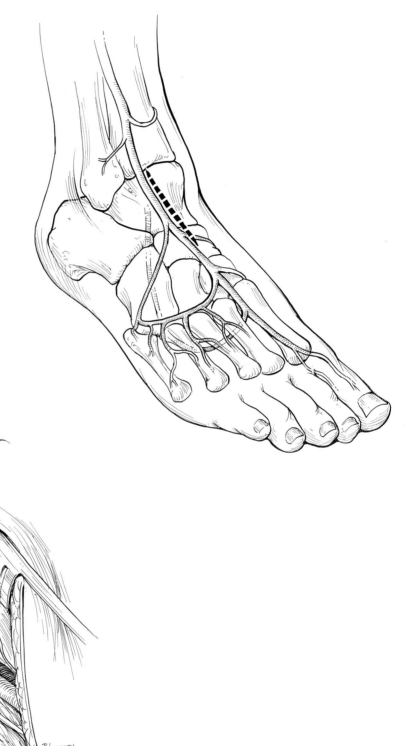

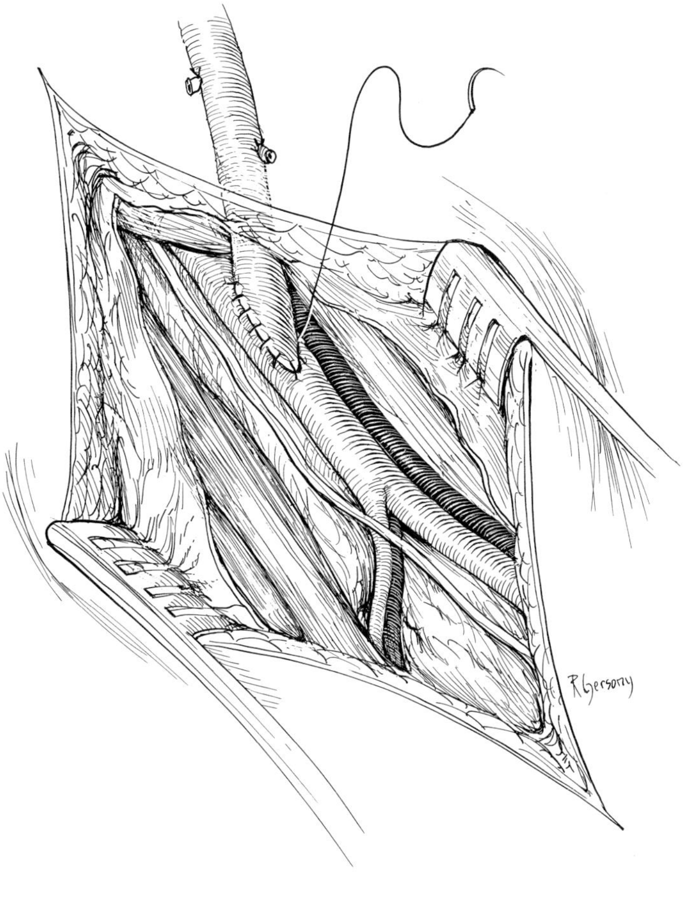

## Figure 40

The distal anastomosis is constructed under tourniquet control using 7-0 polypropylene suture.

# CHAPTER 5

# Femoral Infrapopliteal Bypass With Contralateral Saphenous Vein

Bypass to the infrapopliteal vessels occasionally is necessary when there is no adequate ipsilateral greater saphenous vein. Whereas prosthetic bypass grafting to the above-knee popliteal and below-knee popliteal outflow is associated with acceptable long-term patency, the relatively poor results of prosthetic bypass to the crural arteries make this alternative less desirable. A variety of alternative conduits exist, including arm vein and lesser saphenous vein, but the best option, if available, is the contralateral greater saphenous vein. Preoperative vein mapping assists in determining whether the vein is adequate. If significant contralateral arterial occlusive disease or a popliteal aneurysm exists, options other than the contralateral vein should be considered.

## OPERATIVE PROCEDURE

After the decision to perform a bypass with contralateral saphenous vein has been made, the patient is placed in the supine position with the leg abducted and externally rotated on the "donor" side. The "recipient" leg is internally rotated as needed to facilitate exposure of the anterior tibial artery or the lateral approach to the peroneal artery. Conversely, the recipient leg is externally rotated to expose the posterior tibial artery or to expose the peroneal artery from the medial approach.

A suitable length of vein is harvested though a single, long incision or multiple bridged incisions. The ipsilateral common femoral artery is exposed, as is the crural outflow vessel. In the case of bypass to the anterior tibial artery and when using the lateral approach to the peroneal artery, a lateral subcutaneous tunnel lessens the length of vein necessary to bridge the gap. We often approach the anterior tibial artery in this manner, attempting to place the site of distal anastomosis within the distal one half of the leg. More proximal exposure of the anterior tibial artery is also feasible, but the artery is much deeper there as a result of the large muscle bellies in the proximal calf. We usually approach the peroneal artery medially, except in repeated peroneal bypasses, in which this exposure is obscured by dense scar formation.

A nonreversed vein orientation is advantageous when marked discrepancies exist in the diameter of the two ends of the vein. Figure 41 illustrates the sites of incision for harvest of contralateral greater saphenous vein and the lateral exposure of the peroneal artery with fibular resection. The peroneal artery lies immediately deep to the fibula, and care is taken to avoid injury to the artery and surrounding veins during resection of the bone.

Circumferential exposure of crural vessels may be associated with arterial spasm and troublesome venous bleeding. The use of an occluding tourniquet during performance of the distal anastomosis obviates this problem, requiring exposure of only a narrow strip of the superficial aspect of the vessel.

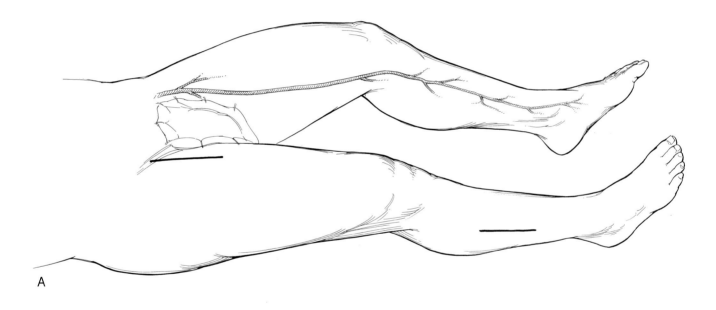

A

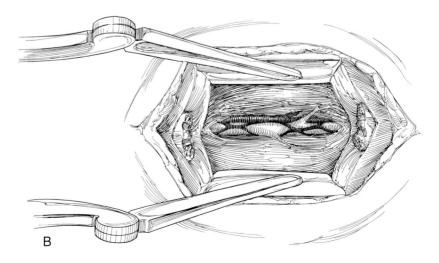

B

## Figure 41

*A,* The contralateral leg is externally rotated to facilitate harvest of the saphenous vein. The ipsilateral leg is internally rotated to bring the lateral calf into view and aid in the lateral exposure of the peroneal artery. *B,* The peroneal incision is placed directly over the fibula. The fibula is circumferentially cleared of adherent tissue with a periosteal elevator, taking care to avoid injury to the peroneal vessels lying immediately deep to the bone. A short length of fibula is resected with bone shears, and the artery is exposed.

### Femoral Infrapopliteal Bypass With Contralateral Saphenous Vein

The patient is administered heparin, and the femoral bifurcation vessels are occluded. After completion of the proximal anastomosis with 6-0 polypropylene suture, the flow through the graft is checked visually (Fig. 42). The graft is tunneled in a lateral subcutaneous space, crossing the knee at a mid-flexion point (Fig. 43). Placing the vein below the iliotibial tract at the level of the knee leads to kinking during knee flexion and early failure of the graft. Similarly, the graft may be compromised if it is tunneled too far anteriorly or posteriorly.

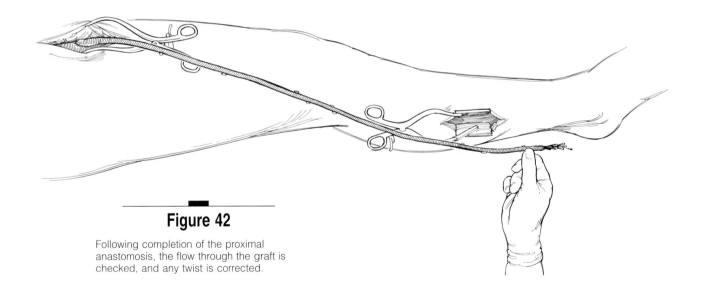

**Figure 42**

Following completion of the proximal anastomosis, the flow through the graft is checked, and any twist is corrected.

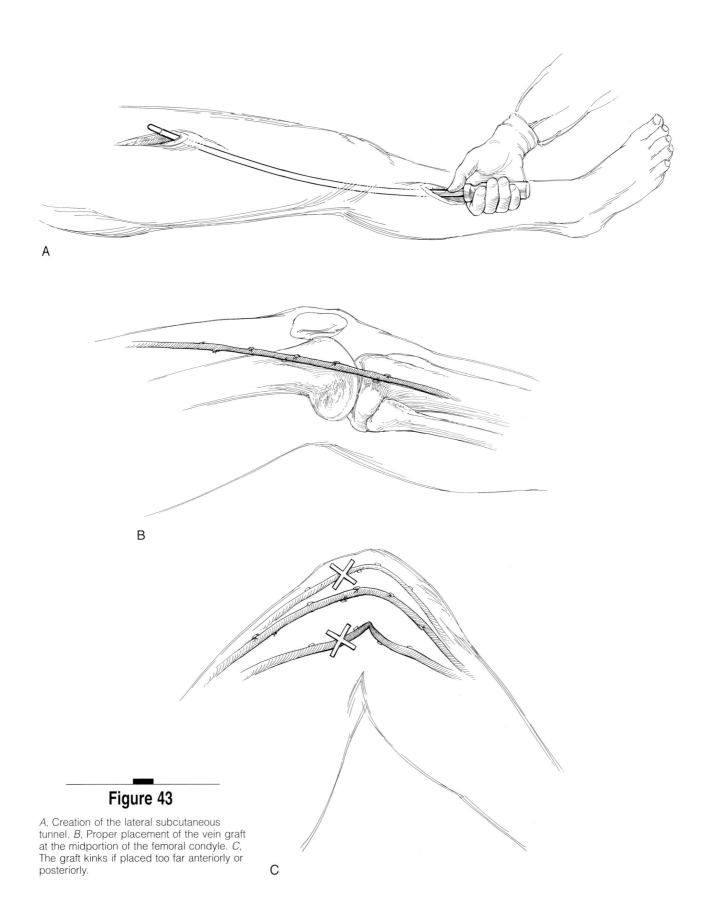

## Figure 43

*A,* Creation of the lateral subcutaneous
tunnel. *B,* Proper placement of the vein graft
at the midportion of the femoral condyle. *C,*
The graft kinks if placed too far anteriorly or
posteriorly.

## *Femoral Infrapopliteal Bypass With Contralateral Saphenous Vein*

Flow through the graft is checked once more by releasing its outflow after it has been tunneled to the distal wound. A sterile tourniquet is placed over a wrap of protective gauze, immediately proximal to the distal incision, to minimize the amount of venous backbleeding into the arterial anastomosis. An Esmarch bandage is applied (Fig. 44), and the tourniquet is inflated (Fig. 45). Complete occlusion of arterial inflow must be ensured before making the tibial arteriotomy, and calcific vascular wall changes associated with diabetic arterial disease may force the operator to raise the level of the tourniquet to a more proximal level, such as the low or high regions of the thigh. The Doppler probe is helpful in ascertaining whether complete inflow occlusion has been achieved by listening for crural flow after inflation of the tourniquet.

The crural artery is palpated to locate a soft segment suitable for anastomosis. An arteriotomy is made, taking care not to injure the back wall of the vessel with the knife blade. The arteriotomy is extended with fine Potts scissors, and the distal anastomosis is completed with 7-0 polypropylene suture (Fig. 46).

Gentle digital pressure is kept on the outflow vessel during release of the tourniquet to prevent air from entering the distal arterial bed. The graft and the adjoining arterial vessels are assessed with Doppler ultrasonography, intraoperative duplex scanning, or arteriography. The graft is interrogated for flow characteristics (e.g., sufficient velocity of blood flow velocity, absence of stenotic lesions), the anastomoses are evaluated with regard to technical problems, and the inflow and outflow vessels are checked for clamp injury or spasm. Heparin may or may not be reversed with protamine sulfate, depending on the adequacy of hemostasis and the operating surgeon's confidence in the reconstruction. The incisions are closed with subcutaneous running absorbable suture to minimize lymphatic leak, and the skin is closed with running absorbable subcuticular suture, interrupted nylon vertical mattress sutures, or clips.

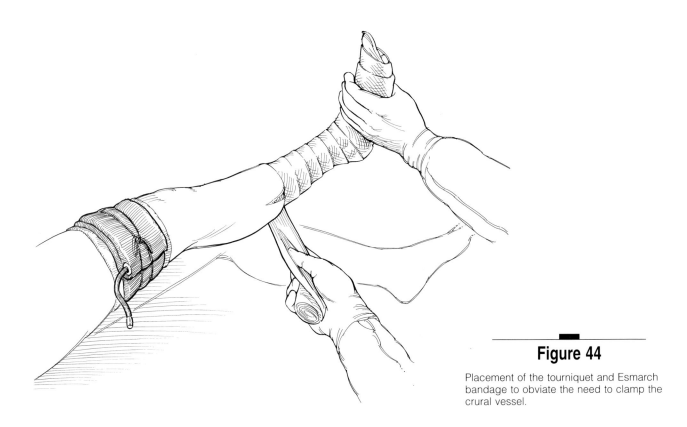

### Figure 44

Placement of the tourniquet and Esmarch bandage to obviate the need to clamp the crural vessel.

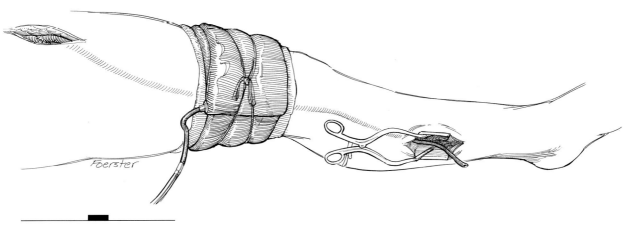

**Figure 45**

Exposure for construction of the distal
anastomosis.

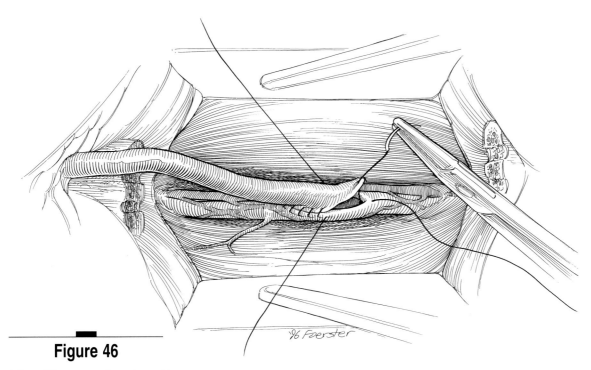

**Figure 46**

Completion of the peroneal anastomosis
with a two-stitch technique.

# CHAPTER 6

# *Profunda Femoris Inflow for Infrainguinal Bypass*

The profunda femoris artery can be an excellent inflow alternative to the common femoral artery in certain situations. The clinical settings for which profunda inflow may be desirable include a hostile groin from multiple previous procedures or inflammation, a calcific but nonstenotic common femoral bifurcation, and a limited length of usable autogenous vein available to reach the closest suitable distal outflow site.

## OPERATIVE PROCEDURE

Exposure of the profunda femoris artery begins well below the groin crease, approaching the middle third of the vessel beyond its first few large muscular branches (Fig. 47). The incision is made in the crease between the rectus femoris and sartorius muscles. The sartorius muscle is retracted medially while the rectus femoris and the vastus medialis muscles are retracted laterally (Fig. 48). The superficial femoral vascular bundle, lying directly below the sartorius, is freed for a distance of several centimeters and retracted medially. Care should be exercised to avoid injury to the terminal branches of the femoral nerve running lateral to the superficial femoral artery.

Palpation of the femur is the key to locating the profunda femoris artery. It lies deep at the bottom of a valley formed by the vastus medialis and the adductor longus and below their strong investing fascial bridge. The profunda is located 1 or 2 cm medial to the femur in the upper thigh, but it assumes a deeper and more lateral location as it courses distally. When a distal incision has been employed at the level of the mid-thigh, the profunda is found in juxtaposition to the medial surface of the femur. In difficult cases, a Doppler instrument may assist in locating the profunda.

After the overlying veins are mobilized, muscular branches of the profunda are controlled with Silastic vessel loops or suture, and smaller branches are ligated and divided. The outflow vessel is then exposed. After adequate heparinization, the proximal anastomosis is performed with 6-0 polypropylene suture.

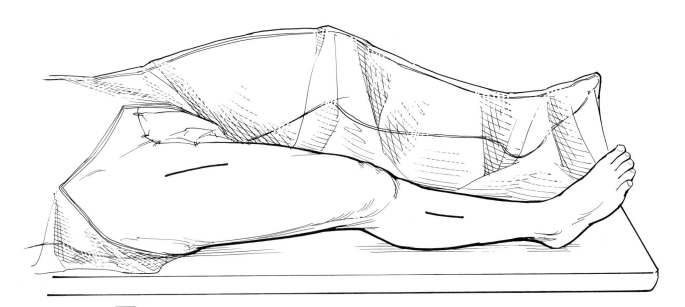

**Figure 47**

Incisions used for a bypass originating from
the profunda femoris artery and terminating
on the anterior tibial artery. Harvest of the
conduit is not illustrated but could be an
arm vein, contralateral greater saphenous
vein, or lesser saphenous vein.

## Profunda Femoris Inflow for Infrainguinal Bypass

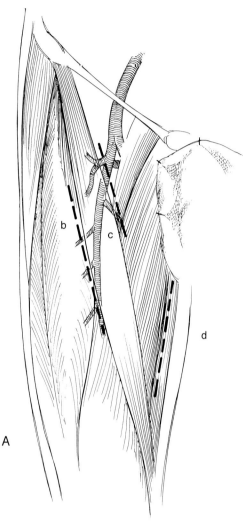

A

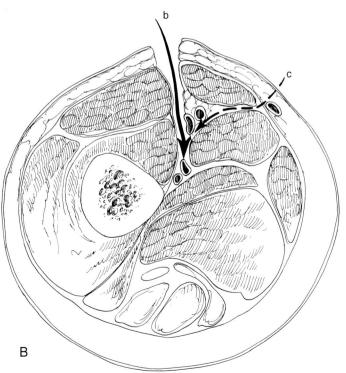

B

### Figure 48

*A,* Three different incisions (marked b, c, and d) can be used to expose the middle and distal thirds of the profunda femoris artery. *B,* A cross-sectional view shows the anterolateral (b) and anteromedial (c) approaches, passing lateral and medial to the sartorius muscle, respectively, and to one side of the superficial femoral vessels to reach the profunda femoris artery. *C,* After passing deep to the superficial femoral vessels, between the vastus medialis and the adductor longus muscles, a raphe is found barring the way to the profunda femoris vessels. *D,* When this raphe is incised, the profunda femoris vessels are encountered, with the vein uppermost. *E,* After dividing a few branches of the adjacent vein, the profunda femoris artery can be exposed and controlled with encircling tapes.

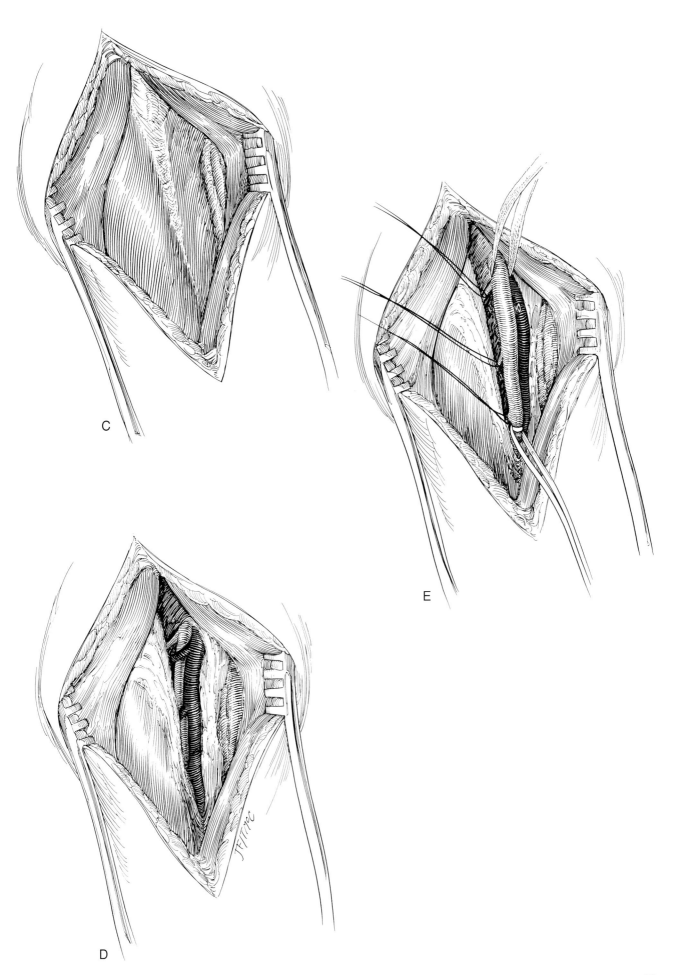

C

D

E

## *Profunda Femoris Inflow for Infrainguinal Bypass*

Figure 49 illustrates the use of autogenous vein that is anastomosed to the profunda femoris artery well below the level of the common femoral bifurcation. The vein is tunneled laterally to the anterior tibial incision (Fig. 50). The crural fascia is incised superiorly to avoid compression of the graft as it turns deep to reach the anterior tibial artery. Flow is checked with the knee flexed. The distal anastomosis is then performed with polypropylene suture, using Silastic vessel loops to control the outflow vessel (Fig. 51) or, more commonly, using an occluding tourniquet.

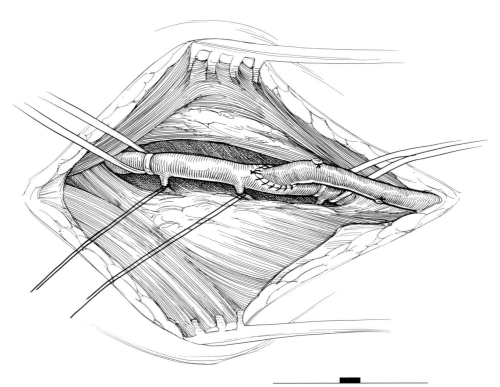

## Figure 49

The completed proximal anastomosis is constructed in an end-to-side fashion with 6-0 polypropylene suture.

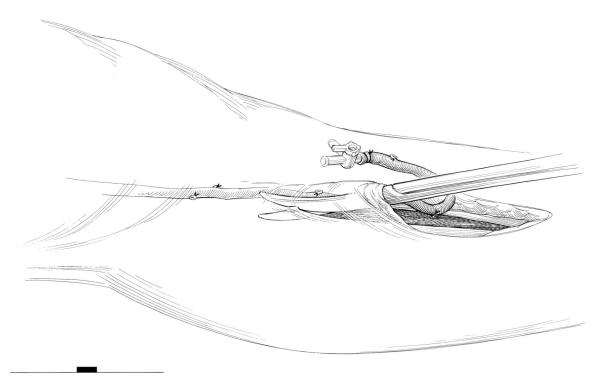

## Figure 50

The anterior compartment fascia is incised
to prevent kinking of the vein graft as it
descends to the anterior tibial artery.

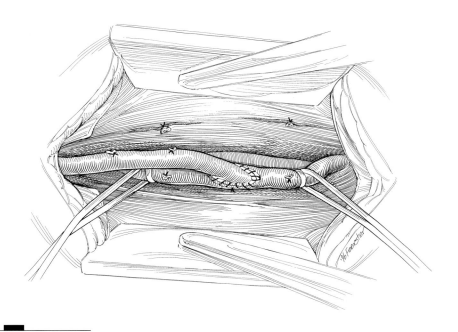

## Figure 51

The distal anastomosis to the anterior tibial
artery is constructed with 7-0 polypropylene
suture.

# CHAPTER 7

# Infrapopliteal Bypass With a Prosthetic Conduit

The results of prosthetic bypasses to the crural vessels are dismally poor. This is not surprising, given the long, large-diameter, and relatively inelastic conduit that, when anastomosed to a tiny artery with high outflow resistance, results in low blood velocity across the foreign luminal surface. If a "critical thrombotic velocity threshold" exists at which graft failure is inevitable, infrapopliteal prosthetic bypass may be the perfect scenario. Moreover, prosthetic grafts are relatively rigid compared with the compliant native artery. Distortion of the anastomosis may occur during systole, because the native artery expands but the graft does not. Repeated localized flexion of the artery may result in vessel wall injury and platelet deposition, contributing to graft failure.

Several technical advances have addressed this problem. The distal arteriovenous (AV) fistula is associated with an increase in graft blood flow, directly addressing the issue of critical thrombotic threshold. Concerns about a steal phenomenon as blood rapidly traverses the long graft have not been borne out; pressure gradients across the graft are infrequently observed. Distal vein cuffs and patches address problems of compliance mismatch and anastomotic distortion, because the venous tissue acts as an intermediary between the noncompliant prosthetic graft and the native artery. Vein collars and patches provide an increased diameter at the area of maximal platelet deposition and intimal hyperplasia, possibly resulting in an improved ability to accommodate these anastomotic changes.

Although the results of prosthetic bypass to crural vessels can never be expected to approach those of autogenous vein bypass, distal anastomotic techniques may improve patency rates to acceptable levels. Critical ischemia in the patient with crural outflow but an inadequate autogenous vein may no longer necessitate primary amputation. Although it has never been proven in a controlled trial, retrospective data suggest that limb viability may be prolonged through the use of a prosthetic bypass with a distal AV fistula or vein patch modification.

# OPERATIVE PROCEDURE

The patient's leg is prepared in the standard fashion, covering the foot with a transparent plastic bag. Complete preparation of the foot, covering the toes with a surgical glove, is necessary when the outflow is to an inframalleolar vessel. The common femoral artery is exposed in the groin, along with a small length of accessory saphenous vein if a distal venous patch is planned. Exposure of the external iliac artery through a transverse incision placed immediately above the inguinal ligament may be an easier option when the groin has been the site of multiple previous bypass procedures, because it avoids the hostile, scarred femoral exposure. Similarly, the distal profunda femoris artery may be used for inflow in repeat procedures.

The crural vessel is exposed, carefully preserving the crural veins so that one may be used in the construction of the AV fistula. A suitable graft, usually a 6-mm, externally supported ePTFE conduit, is tunneled between the two incisions with the aid of a single counterincision placed at the knee level (Fig. 52A). It is advantageous to tunnel the graft below the crural fascia in the lower leg, allowing closure of the fascia over the distal graft and protection of the prosthetic material in case wound disruption occurs. The patient is administered anticoagulants.

A two-team approach allows simultaneous construction of the proximal and distal anastomoses. The femoral anastomosis is constructed in an end-to-side fashion using 6-0 polypropylene or 7-0 Gore-Tex suture (Fig. 52B). The leg is wrapped with an Esmarch bandage, and a tourniquet is placed above the crural wound.

**Construction of a Distal Arteriovenous Fistula.** The crural artery is palpated to find the least diseased segment suitable for anastomosis. The larger of the two crural veins is chosen, and branches are ligated with fine suture to allow close apposition of the artery and vein. Two parallel incisions are made in the vessels, taking care not to injure the opposite wall of the flattened vein with the knife blade (Fig. 52C). The venotomy is approximately two thirds of the length of the arteriotomy, and it is begun slightly distal to the beginning of the arteriotomy so that the heel and toe of the anastomosis lie on the artery alone, allowing the precise placement of sutures at points of arterial outflow.

The ePTFE graft is cut to an appropriate length, and the most distal external supporting rings are removed. The graft is beveled, and the anastomosis is begun with 7-0 polypropylene suture, sewing the back walls of the artery and vein together with a running stitch (Fig. 52D). The ends of the suture are left long, allowing them to be tied to the main anastomotic suture subsequently. After the posterior suture line is complete, the conjoined artery and vein assume an elliptical shape, similar to a standard arteriotomy in a larger vessel. The graft anastomosis is begun at the heel, taking stitches outside-in on the graft and inside-out on the crural artery, and sliding the graft down to the artery in a "parachute" fashion after placement of two to three sutures on each side. Running the single suture around the toe and tying the suture at the midportion of the anastomosis

### Infrapopliteal Bypass With a Prosthetic Conduit

(Fig. 52*E*) completes the anastomosis. Alternatively, a two-suture technique is advisable when visualization at the anastomotic toe is poor.

Intraoperative duplex scanning or contrast arteriography is performed to ensure the technical adequacy of the reconstruction. We prefer the former, because preferential filling of contrast into the vein precludes adequate imaging of the arterial outflow with the latter method. Heparin may or may not be reversed with protamine sulfate. The wounds are closed in layers, and the patient is begun on long-term warfarin anticoagulation.

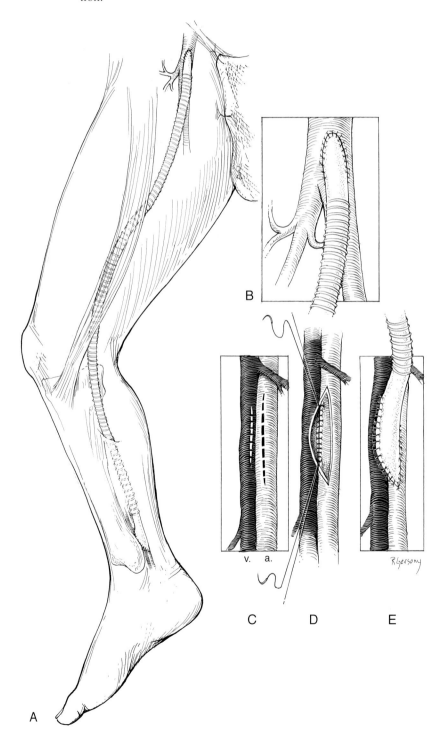

### Figure 52

*A*, Placement of a femoral to posterior tibial, externally supported ePTFE conduit using a single counterincision at the level of the knee. *B*, Construction of the femoral anastomosis with polypropylene or Gore-Tex suture. *C*, Under tourniquet control, small venous branches are ligated, and parallel arterial and venous incisions are made. The venous incision is approximately two thirds the length of the arteriotomy to allow accurate placement of sutures at the toe and heel of the anastomosis. *D*, The back row of the arteriovenous fistula is completed with 7-0 polypropylene suture. *E*, The graft is sutured over the conjoined artery and vein using 7-0 polypropylene suture.

**Construction of a Taylor Patch.** Linton first described the use of a vein patch when an outflow artery was severely diseased. The patch is sutured over the arteriotomy, and the bypass graft then is anastomosed to the patch instead of the artery. Seigman and, later, Miller described the use of a "collar" or "cuff" of vein to provide a smooth transition between a relatively rigid prosthesis and the native artery. After observing a decrease in intimal hyperplasia when a vein extension had been anastomosed to an ePTFE graft, Taylor began to "patch" the distal anastomoses of prosthetic infragenicular reconstructions with a piece of autogenous vein.

In this latter technique, the distal anastomosis is begun by removing the external rings from the last few centimeters of the ePTFE graft. A long arteriotomy is made; it is at least 3 cm long. The graft is cut to the appropriate length, and the end is beveled slightly, excising a U-shaped slit from the hood (Fig. 53). The heel of the anastomosis is constructed with 7-0 polypropylene or ePTFE suture, placing the stitches in a parachute fashion and completing the running suture line to the ends of the prosthetic material. A segment of vein, harvested from the leg or arm, is used as a patch to close the remaining diamond-shaped defect (Fig. 54). Approximately one third of the length of the arteriotomy is composed of prosthetic graft and two thirds of vein patch. Postoperatively, the patient is begun on warfarin in an effort to improve the long-term patency of the reconstruction.

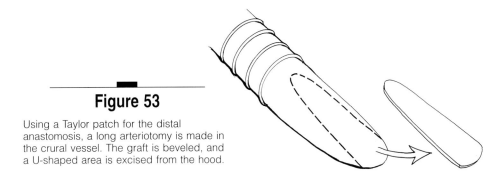

**Figure 53**

Using a Taylor patch for the distal anastomosis, a long arteriotomy is made in the crural vessel. The graft is beveled, and a U-shaped area is excised from the hood.

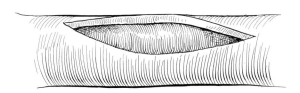

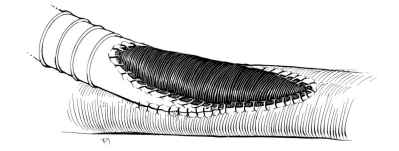

**Figure 54**

The prosthetic graft is sewn to the heel of the anastomosis, and the remainder is completed with a venous patch. When completed, the vein patch forms most of the luminal surface of the anastomotic hood.

# CHAPTER 8

# *Popliteal-Crural Bypass Through the Posterior Approach*

Atherosclerotic occlusive disease of the proximal crural vessels is a common pattern observed in the diabetic population and is associated with limb-threatening ischemia, even in the absence of tandem proximal occlusive lesions. Operative revascularization, using autogenous vein grafts to bridge the gap between the normal popliteal inflow and a patent crural vessel, represents the mainstay of treatment.

The standard approach to infragenicular reconstruction involves a medial approach, gaining access to the inflow and outflow vessels through the same incision used for harvest of the saphenous venous conduit. However, several limitations of this standard technique exist. First, exposure of the proximal portions of the tibial arteries is arduous, primarily as a result of the bulky proximal calf muscles obscuring the vessels. Second, when the greater saphenous vein is absent, harvesting the lesser saphenous vein must be performed through a separate posterior incision, which requires vigorous elevation of the leg by an assistant and the surgeon working while "standing on his head"; complex, indirect harvest techniques; or the use of the prone position during lesser saphenous vein harvest with repositioning thereafter. Third, a medial approach renders exposure of the midportion of the popliteal artery difficult; the medial head of the gastrocnemius muscle overlies this segment and must be divided if access is necessary. Fourth, large areas of ulceration may encompass the area planned for vein harvest or distal arterial exposure, making an alternative approach desirable.

A posterior approach to the popliteal and crural vessels has been described that provides direct access to the lesser saphenous vein, the popliteal artery throughout its course, and all three crural vessels. The procedure preserves the greater saphenous vein and facilitates exposure of the proximal crural vessels, minimizing the required length of venous conduit. The technique is particularly useful in patients with isolated popliteal trifurcation disease, for whom a short bypass can restore normal arterial flow to the foot. Similarly, patients with progression of distal disease after a femoropopliteal bypass are also appropriate candidates for a posterior approach, using lesser saphenous vein to circumvent popliteal and proximal tibial artery stenoses.

All patients should undergo preoperative arteriography with views adequate to visualize the poorly perfused distal vessels. The posterior approach is feasible when the aortoiliac segment, the common femoral artery, and the proximal one half of the superficial femoral artery are free of hemodynamically significant narrowings. The outflow vessel can be any of the three crural vessels or the posterior tibial branches in the foot (i.e., lateral or medial plantar arteries). We have not, however, used the posterior approach for bypasses to the dorsalis pedis artery. The lesser saphenous vein should be mapped with duplex ultrasonography to define its diameter and useable length. The greater saphenous vein may be employed when the lesser saphenous vein is inadequate, and it can be readily harvested, with the patient in the prone position, from the level of the medial malleolus to the mid-thigh.

# OPERATIVE PROCEDURE

General or regional anesthesia is appropriate for most patients, but those with severe chronic obstructive lung disease may not tolerate the prone position under spinal or epidural technique. Whereas the knee joints are mildly flexed during most surgical procedures performed in the prone position, a soft bolster is placed beneath the ipsilateral knee to bring the leg into full extension for a popliteal-crural bypass. The leg is circumferentially prepared to the level of the buttocks, and the foot is covered with a transparent plastic bag or is prepared completely when the outflow is an inframalleolar vessel.

The operation commences with exposure of the lesser saphenous vein through an uninterrupted incision begun at the level of the mid-calf or lateral malleolus, depending on the length of vein deemed necessary (Fig. 55). Preoperative marking of the vein with the use of duplex scanning can assist in locating the vein, especially in patients with multiple, parallel lesser saphenous systems. The lesser saphenous vein runs beneath the investing deep fascia of the proximal calf, and an unexpected length of vein may be harvested in many patients in whom the vein joins the popliteal vein well above the level of the knee joint.

It is wise to incise the skin in a gentle S shape where the posterior skin crease is crossed to prevent the formation of hypertrophic scar. The lesser saphenous vein may be used in a reversed, in situ, or nonreversed (i.e., valves disrupted) fashion. The greater saphenous vein can be harvested from the prone position in a patient without an adequate lesser saphenous vein. The vein is located just anterior to the medial malleolus and can be followed to the level of the mid-thigh. The greater saphenous vein conduit may be employed in a reversed or nonreversed fashion for a posterior popliteal-crural bypass.

The infragenicular popliteal artery is exposed through the same incision used for lesser saphenous vein harvest, between the two heads of the gastrocnemius muscle (Fig. 56). When the supragenicular popliteal artery must be used for inflow, the incision is extended cranially in a gentle S shape, and the vessel is located as it exits from the adductor canal. Occasionally, the superficial femoral artery must be used for inflow. A separate exposure is used in these cases, making a skin incision over the groove between the sartorius and gracilis muscles at the junction of the middle and lower thirds of the thigh (Fig. 57). The artery is located beneath the sartorius, and its pulse is easily palpated after the anterior retraction of the muscle. In this manner, all but the proximal half of the superficial femoral artery can be exposed from a posterior approach.

## Popliteal-Crural Bypass Through the Posterior Approach

### Figure 55

The lesser saphenous vein is harvested through a longitudinal incision running along the midline of the posterior calf. The incision curves laterally at its inferior aspect, following the vein toward the lateral malleolus. The incision makes a gentle S-shape when the popliteal skin crease is crossed to prevent painful contraction of the scar.

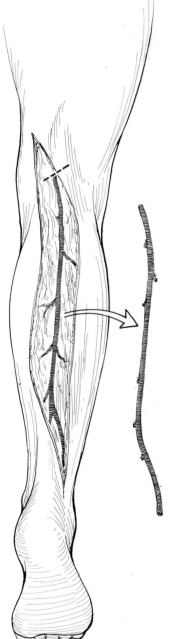

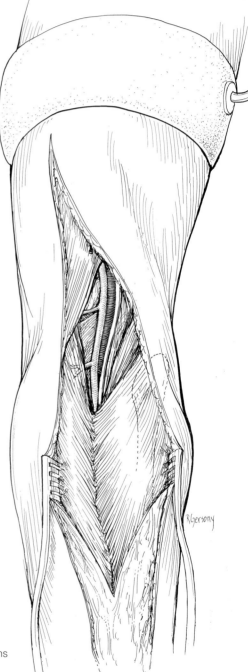

### Figure 56

The midportion of the popliteal artery is exposed between the heads of the gastrocnemius muscle. The crossing veins and the tibial nerve should be carefully avoided.

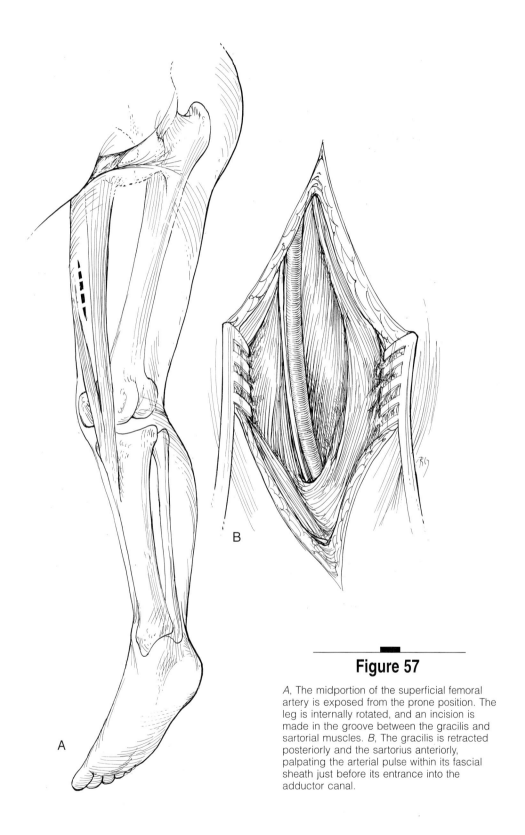

**Figure 57**

*A*, The midportion of the superficial femoral artery is exposed from the prone position. The leg is internally rotated, and an incision is made in the groove between the gracilis and sartorial muscles. *B*, The gracilis is retracted posteriorly and the sartorius anteriorly, palpating the arterial pulse within its fascial sheath just before its entrance into the adductor canal.

### Popliteal-Crural Bypass Through the Posterior Approach

The proximal three crural arteries are exposed by following the popliteal artery to its terminus, lysing the posterior midline fusion of the gastrocnemius heads, and incising the medial aspect of the soleus muscle from its tibial origin (Fig. 58). The lattice of crossing veins should be carefully avoided, as must the diagonally oriented muscular branches of the tibial nerve. The cranial portion of the soleus muscle must be divided to expose the proximal portions of the peroneal and posterior tibial vessels. The anterior

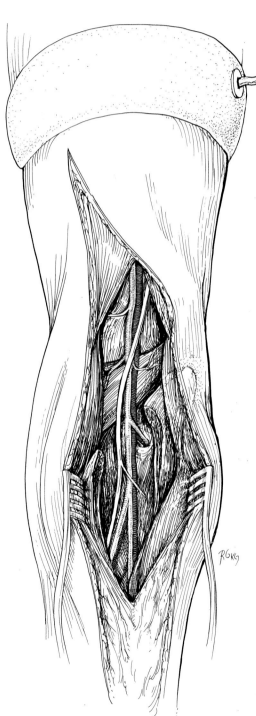

## Figure 58

When disease is limited to the distal popliteal artery, a short bypass to the proximal crural vessel is appropriate. Each of the three crural arteries is exposed by following the popliteal artery distally. The anterior tibial artery, coursing laterally and anteriorly to pierce the interosseus membrane, is easily seen with gentle retraction of the heads of the gastrocnemius muscle. The peroneal and posterior tibial arteries are exposed after incising the junction of the heads of the gastrocnemius muscle and cutting the soleus from its attachment to the tibia. Care must be exercised to avoid injury to the tibial nerve and its branches.

tibial artery is accessible for a distance of 1 or 2 cm before it pierces the interosseous membrane on its anterolateral course. Division of the interosseous membrane provides an additional few centimeters of anterior tibial exposure, but the artery rapidly retreats from view as a result of its curvilinear anterolateral route.

After adequate heparinization, the inflow vessel is clamped. A thigh tourniquet can be employed in cases with severe popliteal calcification that precludes safe clamping of the vessel. Figure 59 illustrates the lesser saphenous vein used in a nonreversed fashion, with the mid-popliteal anastomosis completed with 6-0 polypropylene suture. The valves are sequentially lysed with a Mills valvulotome (Figure 59, *inset*), taking care to avoid inadvertent entry of the valvulotome into the side branches of the vein. Flow through

## Figure 59

The proximal anastomosis is performed to the popliteal artery using a thigh tourniquet to avoid clamping the somewhat diseased vessel. The vein is used in a nonreversed fashion, incising the valves with the Mills valvulotome under the pulsatile pressure of the blood *(inset)*.

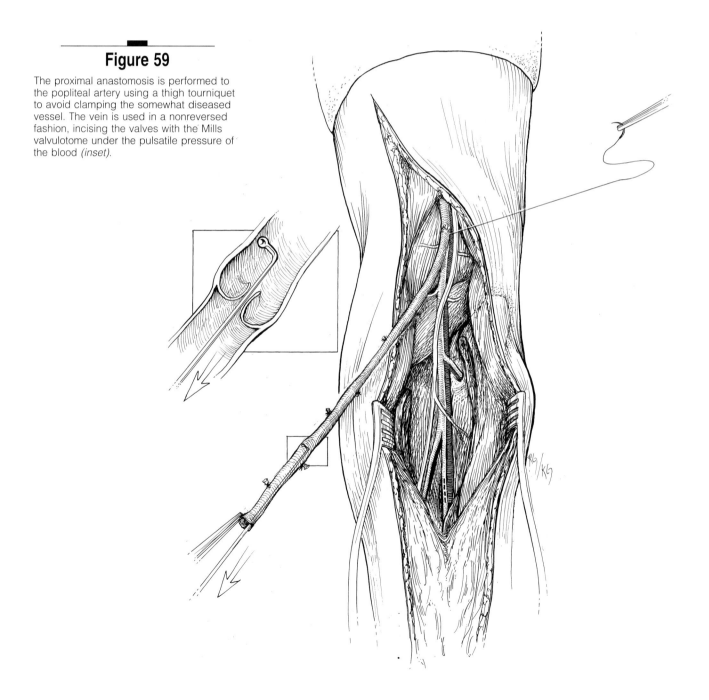

## Popliteal-Crural Bypass Through the Posterior Approach

the vein is assessed visually to ensure adequacy of valve disruption and to be certain that the graft is not twisted. The distal anastomosis is performed to the proximal portion of any one of the three crural arteries. Figure 60 illustrates an anastomosis to the peroneal artery.

Exposure of the outflow vessels below the soleus and gastrocnemius muscle bellies, at the level of the calcaneal tendon, avoids the deep dissection involved with exposure of the proximal crural arteries. An adequate length of autogenous vein allows anastomosis to any of the three distal crural vessels.

The distal posterior tibial artery is exposed in the lower third of the calf. Through the lesser saphenous vein harvest incision, the posterior investing deep fascia of the calf is incised longitudinally, medial to the bulk of the calcaneal tendon within the distal one third of the calf (Fig. 61). The posterior tibial artery is located with medial retraction of

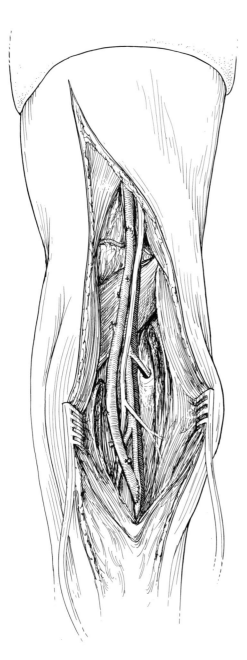

## Figure 60

The tourniquet is reinflated, and the distal anastomosis is performed to the peroneal artery using 7-0 polypropylene suture.

the flexor digitorum longus muscle and lateral retraction of calcaneal tendon. The approach is facilitated with the use of a self-retaining retractor, exposing a long length of the rather superficial distal posterior tibial artery for construction of the anastomosis with 7-0 polypropylene suture. Exposure of the posterior tibial bifurcation, when necessary, is performed through a separate incision placed just posterior to the medial malleolus. The lateral and medial plantar branches can be followed into the foot, an exposure that is facilitated by having the patient in the prone position.

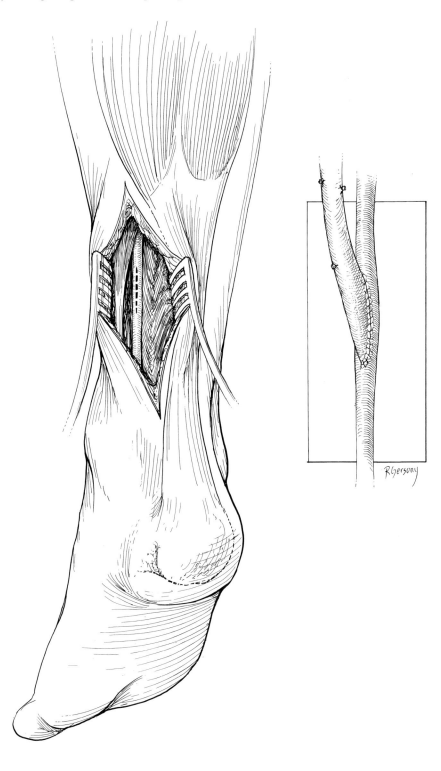

**Figure 61**

More extensive crural artery disease mandates a longer bypass graft to the distal outflow vessels. The lower one third of the posterior tibial artery is exposed in the groove between the flexor digitorum longus and the calcaneal tendon, and the anastomosis is performed with 7-0 polypropylene suture under tourniquet control *(inset).*

## *Popliteal-Crural Bypass Through the Posterior Approach*

The distal peroneal artery is also exposed through the caudal portion of the lesser saphenous vein harvest incision (Fig. 62). The investing deep fascia is incised longitudinally. The calcaneal tendon is retracted medially, with lateral retraction of the flexor hallucis longus muscle. The bony fibula serves as a landmark for the peroneal artery, which may be exposed for a considerable distance before it bifurcates into its anterolateral and posteromedial collateral branches that run to the anterior and posterior tibial arteries, respectively. The anastomosis is completed with 7-0 polypropylene suture under tourniquet control.

The distal anterior tibial artery cannot be easily exposed through the lesser saphenous vein harvest incision. The vessel is approached through an incision identical to that used in the standard, supine technique. The leg is externally rotated to bring the cleft between the anterior tibial and extensor hallucis longus muscles into an accessible orientation. The vein is tunneled from the popliteal fossa to the anterior tibial artery by traversing through the interosseous membrane or, if adequate length is available, through the subcutaneous space around the fibula.

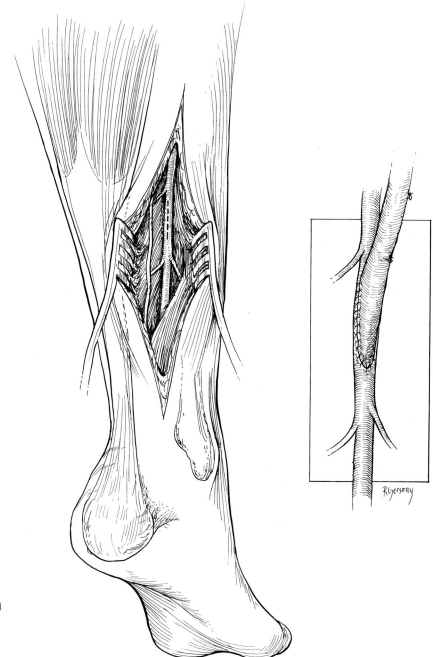

**Figure 62**

The distal peroneal artery is exposed by retracting the calcaneal tendon medially and the flexor hallucis longus tendon laterally. The anastomosis is completed with 7-0 polypropylene *(inset)*.

# OPERATIONS FOR AORTOILIAC OCCLUSIVE DISEASE

# CHAPTER 9

# Aortobifemoral Bypass for Occlusive Disease

Bypass from the aorta to the femoral arteries using a prosthetic graft has been the standard treatment for patients with aortoiliac occlusive disease since the 1960s. Aorto-iliac endarterectomy has played a less important role in the treatment of patients with inflow disease, because the durability of the procedure is poor unless the extent of atherosclerotic disease is limited. Aortoiliac bypass, although obviating the need for groin incisions, is associated with inferior patency rates in patients with concurrent infrainguinal occlusive disease. The procedure presumes the ability to exonerate the iliofemoral segment of disease on the basis of an anteroposterior arteriographic view. Aortofemoral bypass therefore has become the gold standard and is appropriately the most commonly performed arterial reconstruction for symptomatic aortoiliac occlusive disease.

Despite the safety and efficacy of aortofemoral bypass, it has been predicted that the procedure will be less commonly performed as endovascular strategies are developed to address inflow disease. Although the number of such open reconstructions may decrease, the aortobifemoral bypass graft will remain the standard with which all newer technologies should be compared. The procedure can be performed with minimal blood loss, has a perioperative mortality rate between 2 and 3 percent, and achieves a rate of long-term patency approaching 90 percent. Moreover, many patients with extensive calcific occlusions of the iliac arteries or long occlusions of the aorta itself, as well as younger patients with soft, ulcerated atheromatous disease, are likely to be poor candidates for endovascular techniques.

## OPERATIVE PROCEDURE

The patient is sterilely prepared and draped from the nipples to at least the level of the mid-thighs. It is prudent to circumferentially prepare and drape both legs in case an unexpected infrainguinal construction becomes necessary for any reason, such as an intraoperative thromboembolic complication.

The operation is begun with exposure of the femoral arteries through bilateral groin incisions (Fig. 63A), mobilizing an adequate length of profunda femoris artery to allow placement of the toe of the distal anastomosis over any ostial disease. The disparity between the groin skin crease and the inguinal ligament should not be forgotten in a patient with a large abdominal pannus; the novice typically positions the groin incisions below the groin crease and finds the exposure to be far too distal. A transverse incision placed well above the level of the groin crease may provide superior exposure of the common femoral artery in obese individuals (Fig. 63B).

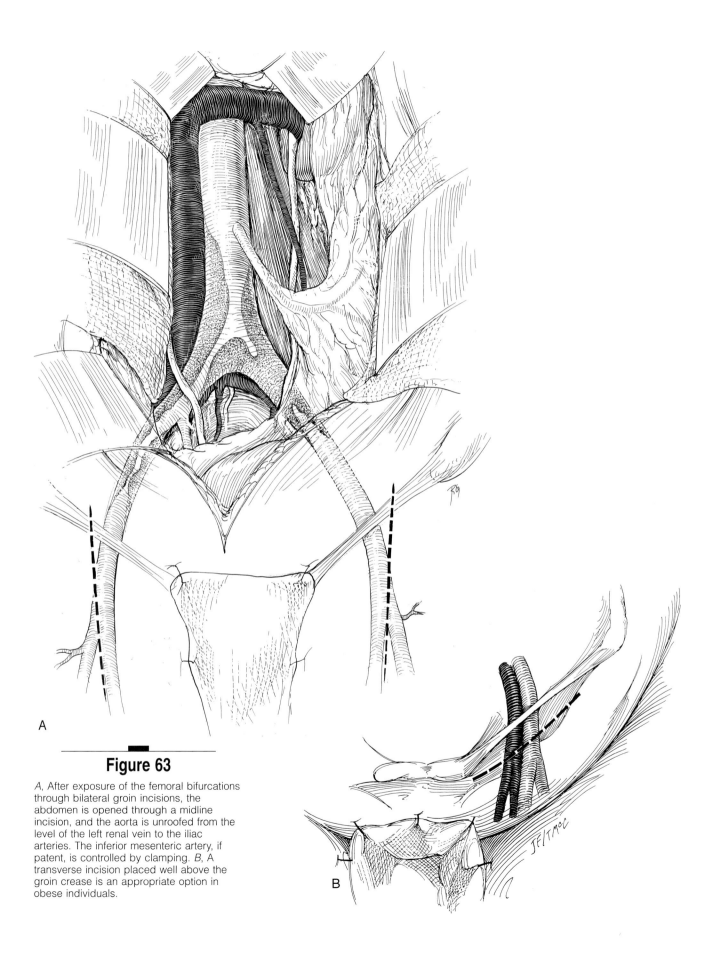

**Figure 63**

*A,* After exposure of the femoral bifurcations through bilateral groin incisions, the abdomen is opened through a midline incision, and the aorta is unroofed from the level of the left renal vein to the iliac arteries. The inferior mesenteric artery, if patent, is controlled by clamping. *B,* A transverse incision placed well above the groin crease is an appropriate option in obese individuals.

## Aortobifemoral Bypass for Occlusive Disease

After exposure and control of the common, superficial, and profunda femoral vessels, the abdomen is opened through a long midline incision. The aorta is exposed with retraction of the small bowel to the right and incision of the retroperitoneum to the left of the duodenum. Circumferential mobilization is not performed until the distal vessels are clamped to avoid distal embolization of atherosclerotic debris.

A Dacron or ePTFE bifurcated graft of suitable size is chosen and retroperitoneal tunnels are created. The tunnels are placed directly anterior to the native iliac arteries, running beneath the ureters. Care must be taken to avoid serious, even life-threatening venous injury during creation of the tunnels. Heparin is administered, and the femoral arteries are clamped to prevent distal embolization. We occlude the inferior mesenteric artery (IMA) at this time, because application of the distal aortic clamp may squeeze aortic debris into the mesenteric circulation. It is only then that the aorta can be safely mobilized circumferentially.

If an end-to-end anastomosis is to be constructed, the lumbar arteries are ligated and divided from the level of the renal vein to the IMA. Care should be taken to avoid injury to lumbar veins crossing beneath the aorta and injury to the occasional retroaortic left renal vein, which is characteristically lower lying than its normal preaortic counter-part.

The aorta is clamped just below the renal arteries and just above the IMA. Placement of the proximal anastomosis below the level of the IMA is unwise because of the more extensive disease in this segment. The aorta is divided, and the distal aortic stump is oversewn with 2-0 or 3-0 polypropylene suture. Alternatively, a vascular stapling device can be used in the rare event that the aorta is pliable at this level.

The body of the graft is cut short (2 to 4 cm), and the proximal anastomosis is constructed with 3-0 polypropylene suture (Fig. 64). If calcific plaque at the proximal anastomosis precludes needle traversal, endarterectomy of an appropriate-length, circular segment of the proximal aortic cuff can be performed. In this case, 5-0 polypropylene suture can be used to lessen needle-hole bleeding from the endarterectomized wall.

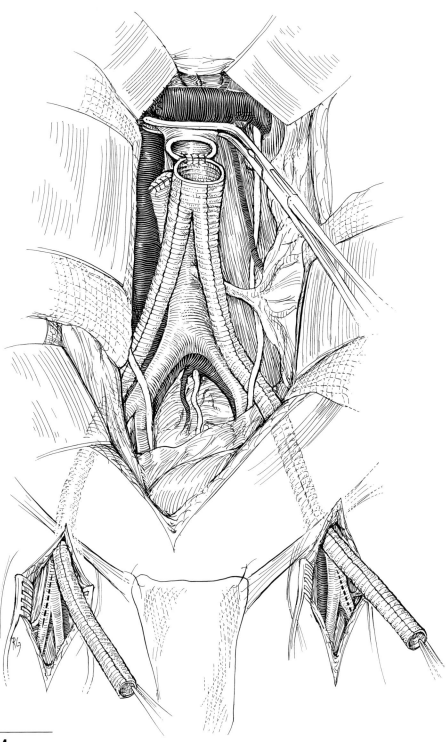

**Figure 64**

The aortic stump is oversewn with stout
polypropylene suture, and the proximal
anastomosis is constructed in an end-to-end
fashion.

## *Aortobifemoral Bypass for Occlusive Disease*

An end-to-side proximal anastomosis is required when retrograde perfusion of patent hypogastric and inferior mesenteric vessels cannot be achieved with an end-to-end procedure and the end-to-side procedure is needed for colon viability or to prevent impotence. The classic instance in which an end-to-side proximal anastomosis is mandatory occurs in the patient with bilateral external iliac artery occlusions. In these cases, a long bevel is placed on the graft to allow an acute angle between the graft and the native aorta (Fig. 65), thereby preventing the body of the graft from rising out of the retroperitoneum at too great an angle after placement. A gentle bevel prevents contact with the bowel or kinking at the graft bifurcation and facilitates closure of the retroperitoneal tissues over the prosthesis. This bevel, however, requires a longer anastomosis.

The aorta is clamped tangentially to obviate the need to disrupt the lumbar arterial flow (Fig. 66). A side-biting clamp is almost never feasible with the thickened aortic wall (Fig. 67). Complete occlusion is rarely achieved with a single side-biting clamp, and visualization of the lumen is inadequate while sewing the anastomosis. With proper technique and exposure, however, construction of an end-to-side proximal anastomosis can be accomplished without difficulty (Fig. 68).

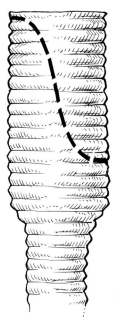

## Figure 65

The body of the graft is beveled in preparation for an end-to-side anastomosis in patients with bilateral external iliac artery occlusive disease.

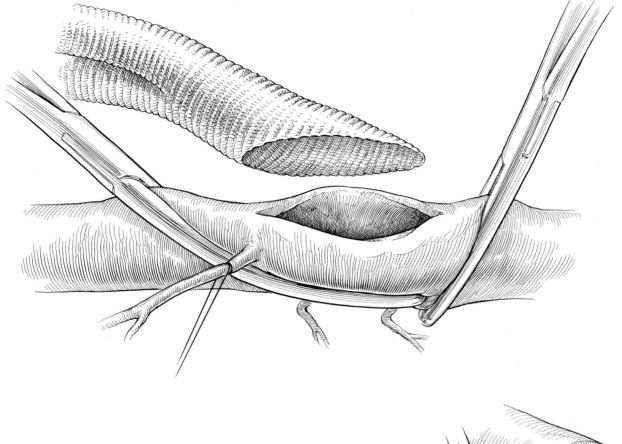

**Figure 66**

Two clamps are used to control the aorta
during the performance of an end-to-side
anastomosis. The lumbar vessels are
controlled without individually exposing
each vessel *(inset)*.

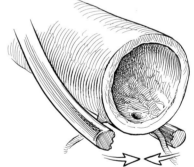

**Figure 67**

A side-biting clamp is seldom appropriate
when clamping the infrarenal aorta.
Adequate control is rarely achieved, and the
thickened aortic wall makes accurate suture
placement difficult.

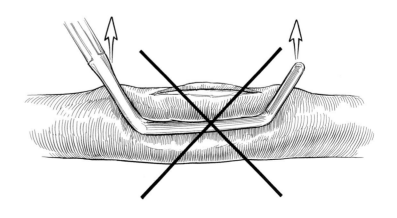

## Aortobifemoral Bypass for Occlusive Disease

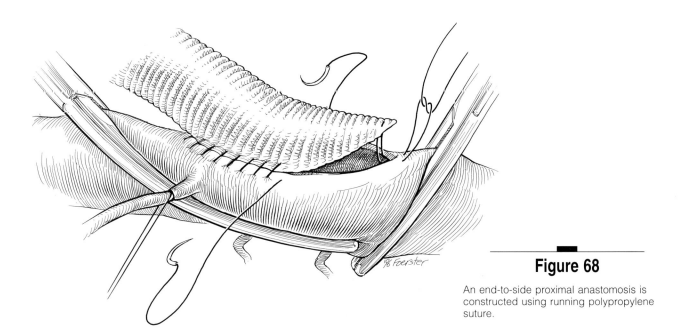

**Figure 68**

An end-to-side proximal anastomosis is constructed using running polypropylene suture.

The distal anastomoses are constructed in an end-to-side fashion, using 5-0 or 6-0 polypropylene suture (Fig. 69). It is usually appropriate to place the toe of distal anastomosis onto the profunda femoris artery, thereby maximizing profunda flow when an unexpected ostial stenosis is present. Carrying the distal anastomosis onto the profunda femoris is particularly important when the superficial femoral artery is occluded.

Air and debris are evacuated from the graft during completion of the anastomoses. The femoral and IMA clamps are released last. Flow through the outflow vessels, including the IMA, is assessed with Doppler or duplex ultrasonography. The feet are assessed for pulses and viability before anticoagulation is reversed with protamine sulfate. The groin wounds are closed in multiple layers to mitigate lymphatic leakage. The graft is retroperitonealized, which occasionally requires the mobilization of a segment of omentum for coverage in thin patients without adequate retroperitoneal tissue. The abdomen is closed in a manner of the operating surgeon's preference.

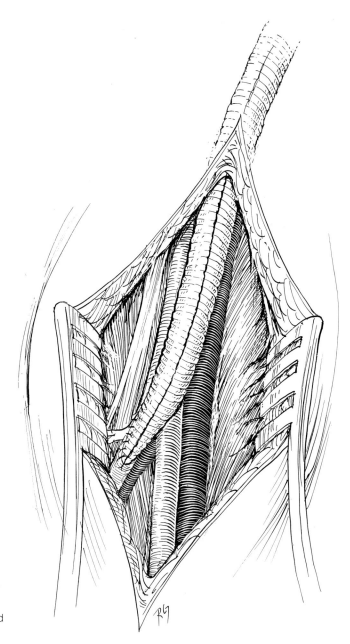

## Figure 69

The distal anastomosis is performed with the toe positioned well onto the profunda femoris artery. In this manner, the anastomosis functions as a patch angioplasty of the commonly encountered profunda ostial stenosis.

# CHAPTER 10

# *Aortoiliac Endarterectomy*

Endarterectomy for aortoiliac occlusive disease was the standard surgical treatment before the advent of reliable, large-diameter prosthetic grafts. The results of early aortoiliac endarterectomy were inferior to those expected today, primarily because the procedure was often performed in patients with extensive aortoiliac occlusive disease extending into the external iliac arteries and even into the femoral system.

Today, aortoiliac endarterectomy is an effective and appropriate procedure when performed in patients with disease limited to the aorta and common iliac arteries. Alternative methods of reconstruction are preferable when the disease extends into the external iliac vessels. Aortofemoral bypass is appropriate for most patients with inflow problems, because a relatively small proportion of patients have the limited extent of disease appropriate for endarterectomy. Moreover, the results of balloon angioplasty with or without intraluminal stenting have lessened the need for this procedure, particularly because candidates for endarterectomy and percutaneous balloon dilatation have a similar anatomic extent of disease.

Nevertheless, aortoiliac endarterectomy in appropriate candidates eliminates an embolic source and restores normal inflow without the need for a prosthetic bypass graft. This feature is important in young persons, whose long life expectancy may result in the need for secondary reconstructive procedures. Younger patients also may have soft atheromatous disease, which is poorly amenable to percutaneous procedures. For these reasons, we remain aggressive in considering aortoiliac endarterectomy for younger patients with such indications and anatomy.

## OPERATIVE PROCEDURE

The patient is widely prepared and draped, including the groin in case an aortofemoral bypass becomes necessary. The procedure is begun with a midline, transabdominal approach to the aorta and iliac vessels (Fig. 70). The proximal external iliac arteries are fully exposed and carefully palpated early in the dissection. Incision of the retroperitoneal reflection lateral to the cecum for the right external iliac artery and to the sigmoid colon for the left iliac arteries aids the exposure in many patients, especially the obese. Identification of disease beyond the origin of the external iliac artery contraindicates the procedure, and an aortofemoral bypass should be performed instead. It is not unusual for a tongue of yellow atherosclerotic plaque to extend into the first 1 or 2 cm of external iliac artery. This extent of disease is not a contraindication to aortoiliac endarterectomy, but more distal disease negatively affects long-term patency.

70

In contrast to bypass, aortoiliac endarterectomy requires extensive dissection and mobilization of the aortoiliac vessels. Circumferential control of each hypogastric artery is necessary, along with the proximal several centimeters of the external iliac arteries. The inferior mesenteric artery is controlled with a Potts looped Silastic band. Each lumbar vessel should be preserved, controlling backbleeding with delicate (e.g., Gregory, Diethrich) bulldog clamps or Silastic vessel loops. Exposure of the middle sacral artery is facilitated by cephalad retraction of the common iliac arteries, usually with an assistant elevating the vessels with two vein retractors (Fig. 71). The risk of catastrophic venous bleeding dictates cautious dissection and retraction in this area.

## Figure 70

The infrarenal aorta and iliac vessels are exposed in their entirety, including careful isolation of each lumbar artery and the inferior mesenteric artery. The proximal external iliac arteries are carefully palpated for disease. Palpable plaque extending beyond the first 1 or 2 cm of the external iliac arteries should dissuade the surgeon from an endarterectomy.

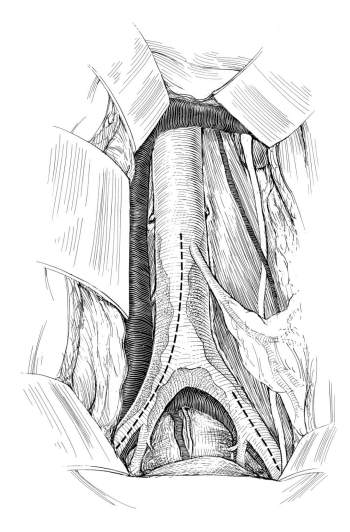

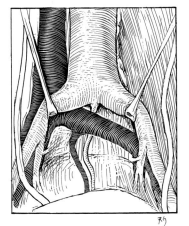

## Figure 71

Cephalad retraction of each common iliac artery with vein retractors provides a means of visualizing and controlling the middle sacral artery.

## Aortoiliac Endarterectomy

Heparin is administered, and the proximal and distal arteries are occluded. Arteriotomies are begun on the distal common iliac vessels and extended distally over the hypogastric orifices (Fig. 72). The feasibility of the procedure can be accurately assessed only at this time, when the adequacy of the endarterectomy end point is evaluated.

Attempts at aortoiliac endarterectomy should be aborted if the endarterectomy cannot be safely ended within 1 or 2 cm of the external iliac origin. In such cases, the arteriotomies should be closed in a manner sufficient to preserve retrograde flow to the hypogastric vessels, and an aortofemoral bypass should be performed.

If the endarterectomies can be ended satisfactorily, the right common iliac arteriotomy is extended onto the aorta and continued to a point above the atherosclerotic plaque. An endarterectomy plane is established, and the plaque is removed with the aid of an endarterectomy spatula. A discontinuous arteriotomy spares the autonomic fibers crossing at the origin of the left common iliac artery. The left common iliac endarterectomy is facilitated through the use of a loop stripper (Fig. 73), but a spatula may suffice if the common iliac artery is relatively short.

The arteriotomies may be closed primarily with 5-0 polypropylene suture, but all but the largest iliac arteries are best closed with an ePTFE or polyester patch (Fig. 74). Postoperative surveillance with Doppler segmental pressure measurements is performed on a regular basis, because thrombosis may be heralded by the development of intimal hyperplastic lesions at the distal endarterectomy sites.

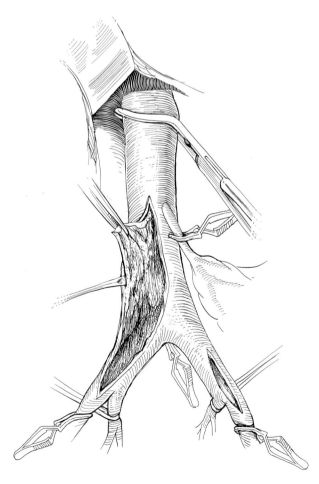

### Figure 72

The vessels are clamped, and a long arteriotomy is made, running from the proximal extent of aortic plaque to the right external iliac artery. A shorter arteriotomy is made over the left hypogastric orifice. An endarterectomy plane is established, and the right iliac plaque and aortic plaque are removed with the aid of an endarterectomy spatula.

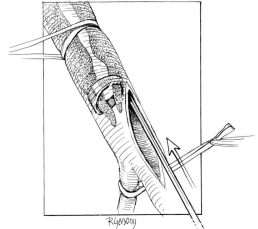

## **Figure 73**

The left iliac endarterectomy is feathered at
the distal end. Using the loop stripper, the
endarterectomy proceeds proximally to
become contiguous with the aortic
specimen.

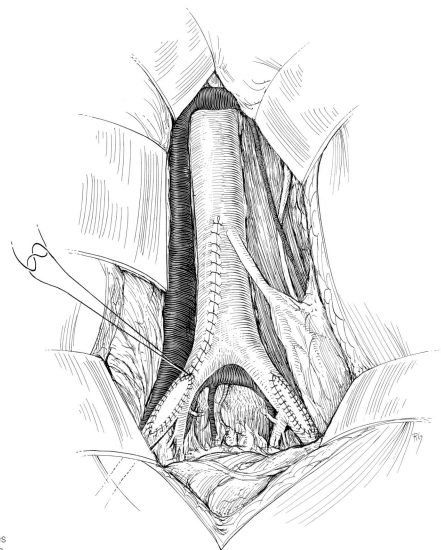

## **Figure 74**

The aortotomy is closed primarily with 5-0
polypropylene suture. The iliac arteriotomies
are closed with ePTFE or polyester patches.

# CHAPTER 11

# Iliofemoral Bypass

In several clinical scenarios, a unilateral "inflow," or suprainguinal, procedure is appropriate for the treatment of aortoiliac occlusive disease. An iliofemoral bypass is an appropriate procedure when the aortic disease is relatively mild and the symptoms are limited to one leg. An iliofemoral bypass may also be a more desirable option than aortobifemoral bypass when a simultaneous infrainguinal reconstruction is planned. The magnitude of the physiologic challenge is less with an iliofemoral bypass, and if necessary, the bypass can be extended to the above-knee popliteal artery with a side-to-side anastomosis to the common femoral or profunda femoris artery.

The femorofemoral bypass is the main competition for iliofemoral bypass. When choosing between the two procedures, the status of the patient must be taken into consideration. Although patency rates may be somewhat higher with an iliofemoral bypass, the procedure is more stressful to the patient. A femorofemoral bypass, however, is inappropriate when the donor iliac segment is stenotic.

Failure to visualize a common iliac stump on the preoperative arteriogram is not an absolute contraindication to iliofemoral bypass. Common iliac arteries occlude as a result of disease at one of two locations. The first group of patients has atherosclerotic disease distally, at the common iliac bifurcation (Fig. 75). This type of patient has a soft, "clampable" proximal iliac artery that can be thrombectomized to serve as an adequate inflow site for an end-to-end proximal anastomosis. The second group of patients suffers common iliac occlusions as a result of atherosclerotic disease proximally, at the common iliac orifice (Fig. 76). This usually represents an extension of severe, distal aortic disease that is difficult to endarterectomize. An attempt at iliofemoral bypass in these patients is fraught with danger, because of the risk of proximal clamp injuries when the rigid arterial wall is disrupted. Although a tapering "beak" of common iliac artery found on preoperative arteriography suggests the presence of proximal iliac atherosclerosis and thus a poor candidate for iliofemoral bypass, we have used preoperative computed tomography scanning to more accurately assess the quality of the proximal common iliac artery to distinguish between these two groups of patients. Iliofemoral bypass should *not* be attempted in patients with dense calcific plaque within the wall of the proximal iliac artery. A femorofemoral or aortofemoral bypass may be more appropriate in these cases.

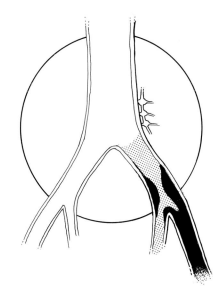

## Figure 75

An iliofemoral bypass is appropriate when the common iliac artery is occluded, as long as the dense atherosclerotic plaque does not extend to the aortic bifurcation.

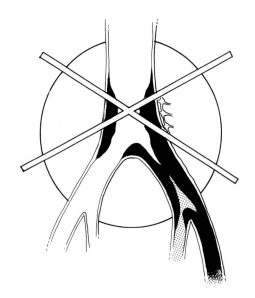

## Figure 76

An iliofemoral bypass is not appropriate when the iliac disease represents a continuation of aortic plaque. Clamp injury to the iliac artery is probable in this instance, resulting in hemorrhage through a crack in the wall of the artery or early occlusion from disruption of the plaque.

*Iliofemoral Bypass*

## OPERATIVE PROCEDURE

General or regional (i.e., spinal or epidural) anesthesia is acceptable for iliofemoral procedures. The patient is placed in the supine position with a roll or bean-bag beneath the ipsilateral flank (Fig. 77). A transverse incision made at the level of the umbilicus runs from the lateral border of the rectus abdominis muscle to a point halfway between the tip of the 12th rib and the iliac crest. The external and internal oblique muscles are divided, and the fibers of the transversus abdominis muscle are bluntly separated. The retroperitoneal space is entered laterally in a plane identified by the yellow fat in this region. A plane is developed between the peritoneal sac and the psoas muscle while retracting the peritoneal contents and ureter medially (Fig. 78). The common and external iliac vessels are easily visualized with this approach, as is the distal aorta (Fig. 79). The proximal anastomosis can be placed on the distal aorta through this exposure if unsuspected severe iliac disease is encountered. The sympathetic chain should be left undisturbed to avoid a bothersome postsympathectomy neuralgia. The femoral bifurcation is exposed through a longitudinal groin incision.

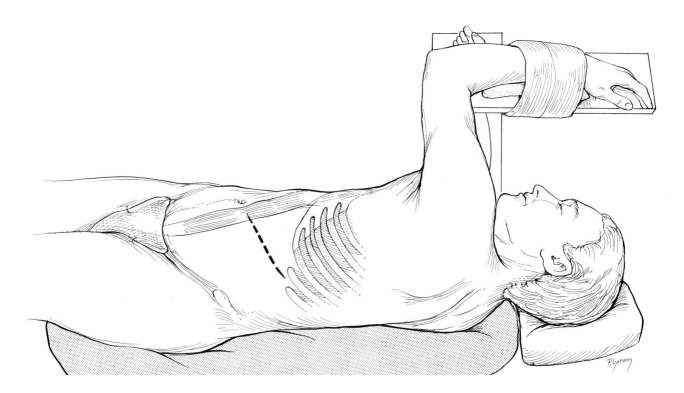

### Figure 77

The patient is positioned with a bolster or beanbag to elevate the flank and spread the space between the iliac crest and the costal margin.

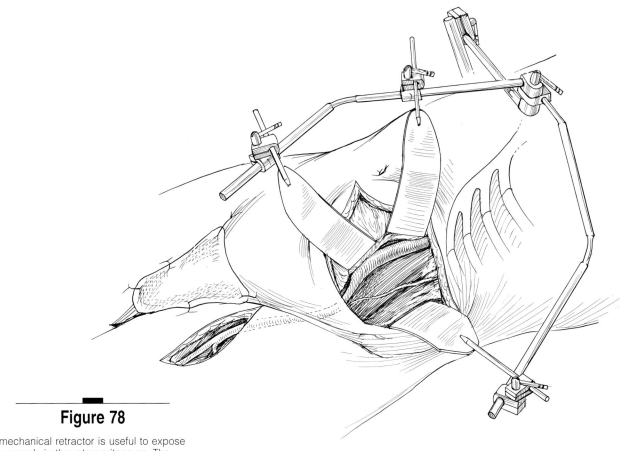

## Figure 78

A mechanical retractor is useful to expose the vessels in the retroperitoneum. The femoral vessels are exposed in the groin.

## Figure 79

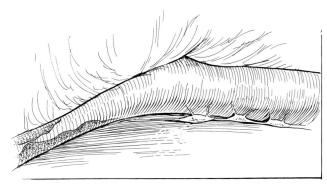

The distal aorta and proximal iliac system are exposed, taking care to avoid injury to the sympathetic chain.

## *Iliofemoral Bypass*

After heparinization, the proximal iliac artery is clamped. If the common iliac artery is occluded, the vessel is transected, and a thrombectomy is performed, restoring inflow with an end-to-end anastomosis. Otherwise, the hypogastric and external iliac vessels are controlled, and a common iliac arteriotomy is made in preparation for an end-to-side anastomosis. Generally, 5-0 polypropylene or Gore-Tex suture is employed. The distal anastomosis is performed to the common femoral artery, with the toe of the anastomosis on the profunda femoris artery (Fig. 80).

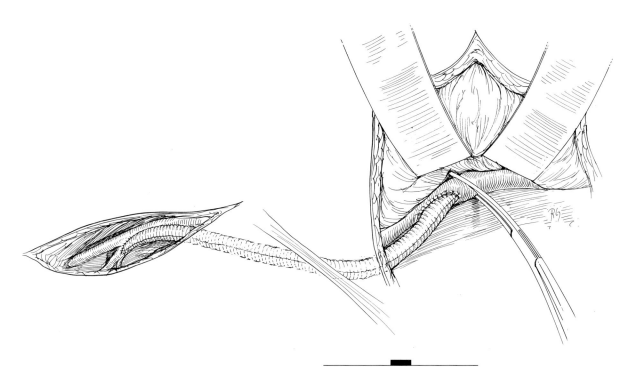

## Figure 80

The completed bypass has an end-to-side proximal anastomosis and a distal anastomosis onto the proximal profunda femoris artery.

# CHAPTER 12

# *Obturator Bypass*

The obturator bypass is a technique used in patients with infected groin wounds, because a route through the obturator space avoids crossing through infected tissue planes. The infectious process often involves the femoral vessels themselves or a graft that terminates there. Occasionally, the procedure can be used when a unilateral groin infection involves only the distal portion of the limb of an aortofemoral graft. A prerequisite for any obturator bypass is that the infection must not have ascended into the retroperitoneum.

An obturator bypass may assume different configurations, depending on the specific choice of inflow and outflow sites. The extent of iliac occlusive disease usually determines whether the proximal anastomosis is placed on the aorta or on the common or external iliac arteries. Conversely, the midportion of an aortobifemoral graft limb may represent an acceptable inflow site if preoperative imaging, intraoperative appearance, and the Gram stain results confirm that the graft infection is limited to the groin. The distal anastomosis of an obturator bypass may be placed on the mid-superficial femoral artery, if it is patent. The above-knee popliteal artery is also an acceptable site. We have found the distal profunda femoris artery to be an ideal site for outflow in patients with superficial femoral occlusion; the artery is exposed through an incision placed at the level of the mid-thigh.

An infected false aneurysm at the proximal anastomosis of a prosthetic femoropopliteal bypass graft is another application for an obturator approach. Excision of the graft and direct repair of the common femoral defect carry a great risk of hemorrhage resulting from breakdown of the repair, especially if the offending organism is virulent. Simple obliterative oversewing of the common femoral artery decreases the risk of subsequent hemorrhage, but leg ischemia is likely from interruption of inflow.

A better alternative is an extra-anatomic bypass of the infected process through uninvolved tissue planes, followed by removal of the graft and oversewing of the common femoral artery. An obturator bypass to the distal profunda femoris artery provides an uninfected route to preserve inflow, allowing subsequent graft excision. If successful, the patient may experience claudication, but the limb will remain viable.

*Obturator Bypass*

## OPERATIVE PROCEDURE

The operation is begun with the patient in a position similar to that for an iliofemoral bypass (Fig. 81). A povidone-iodine–impregnated plastic adherent drape is used to isolate a contaminated groin wound from the clean field. A flank incision is made, and the iliac vessels are exposed (Fig. 82). Sweeping the peritoneal sac from the pelvic floor exposes the obturator foramen, located just below the superior ramus of the pubis. The recipient artery, in this case the distal profunda femoris artery, is exposed through a mid-thigh incision, keeping away from the infected femoropopliteal graft. Creating the tunnel is usually the most arduous part of the procedure. Readjusting the curve of the metallic tunneler to suit the anatomic configuration of the particular patient is usually necessary. The lateral-lying obturator vessels should be specifically avoided when piecing the obturator membrane, because failure to do so results in troublesome bleeding. We generally use an externally supported ePTFE graft to avoid compression or kinking in the inaccessible tunnel (Fig. 83).

Heparin is administered, and the external iliac artery is ligated. The proximal and distal anastomoses are performed in an end-to-side fashion, similar to that described in Chapter 11. After the anastomoses are complete and the wound is tightly closed, an adherent plastic dressing isolates the fresh wounds from contamination during the subsequent part of the operation.

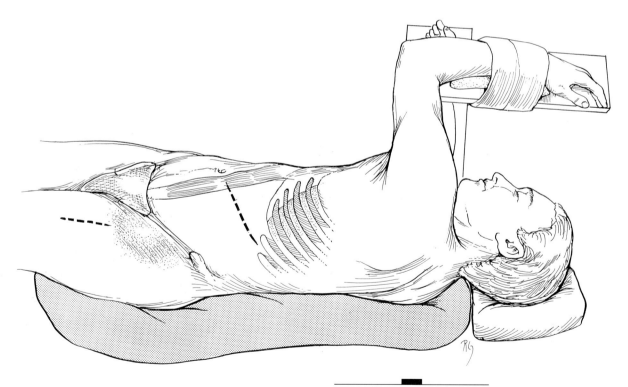

## Figure 81

The patient is positioned with a beanbag supporting the flank in preparation for an obturator bypass.

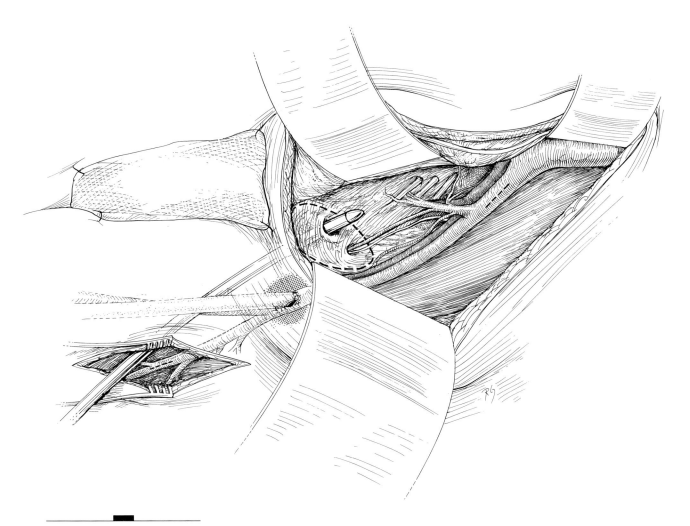

## Figure 82

The retroperitoneal space is entered, and the iliac vessels are identified. The ureter is swept medially with the peritoneal sac. The floor of the pelvis is cleared, and the obturator foramen is identified. The profunda femoris vessel is exposed through an incision placed below the infected groin process. With the tunneler kept well below the groin infection, a tunnel is created between the profunda wound and the retroperitoneum. The obturator membrane is pierced inferior and medial to the obturator vessels, which exit through the obturator foramen at the superolateral aspect of the foramen.

## Obturator Bypass

In the second portion of the procedure, the groin wound is opened, and control of the most proximal aspect of the common femoral artery is obtained. With the bypass in place, profunda backbleeding is vigorously pulsatile. Distal control of the profunda femoris therefore is more critical than proximal control of the common femoral artery, because the external iliac artery was previously ligated. The femoral anastomosis should be addressed only when adequate proximal and distal control has been achieved.

The infected femoropopliteal graft is disconnected from its anastomosis, and the common femoral artery is obliterated with a running 2-0 or 3-0 polypropylene suture. The distal graft anastomosis then is taken down, with the prosthetic material excised in its entirety. The remaining wounds are closed primarily or left open, depending on the virulence of the infectious process. In either case, it is desirable to cover the oversewn common femoral artery with a mobilized flap of sartorius muscle.

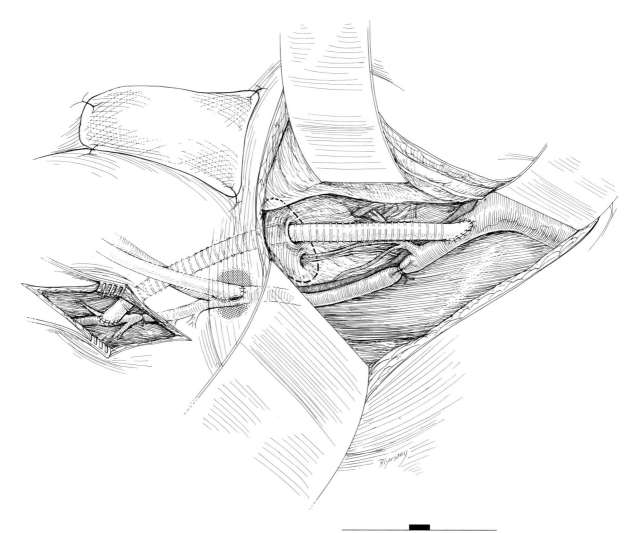

### Figure 83

The external iliac artery is ligated, and the proximal and distal anastomoses of the ringed ePTFE obturator graft are constructed. The old graft is removed after the incisions are closed and sealed.

# CHAPTER 13

# *Femorofemoral Bypass*

A femorofemoral crossover graft is widely employed for bypassing unilateral iliac occlusive disease and is associated with long-term patency rates close to 80 percent in good run-off situations. The prosthetic graft, originating from donor femoral artery, terminates at the femoral artery on the affected side. The procedure is considerably less stressful to the patient than standard aortofemoral bypass, because it avoids an abdominal incision and aortic clamping. Male sexual disturbances, such as retrograde ejaculation from damage to the preaortic sympathetic fibers or impotence from damage to the parasympathetic nervi erigentes at the iliac bifurcations, are not seen with femorofemoral reconstruction. The procedure also provides a relatively simple alternative in the treatment of unilateral aortofemoral graft limb occlusion, avoiding the technical problems associated with reoperative aortic procedures when the occluded graft limb cannot be readily thrombectomized, as is often the case.

Femorofemoral bypass is associated with certain limitations. The procedure puts the contralateral leg at risk if technical misadventures or infection occur at the site of the proximal anastomosis. Of necessity, the donor iliac system must be free of significant stenoses and without significant pressure gradients at rest or with induced hyperemia. Because iliac occlusive disease tends to be bilateral, this requirement limits the applicability of femorofemoral procedures, although the use of adjuvant balloon angioplasty or stenting of a donor iliac artery's stenoses increases the number of eligible patients and does not adversely affect patency.

Placement of a femorofemoral graft in the presence of significant donor iliac disease creates the classic paradigm of the steal phenomenon. The femorofemoral graft increases flow across an occult iliac stenosis, resulting in a drop in perfusion pressure in the donor extremity and the appearance of new symptoms or worsening of existing symptoms in the donor extremity. Biplane arteriography may be used preoperatively to assess the extent of donor iliac occlusive disease, and pressure gradients should be measured as the catheter is withdrawn across the iliac segment. If this has not been done, we measure the common femoral pressure with a needle and transducer at the time of operation. A femorofemoral bypass is inappropriate in the presence of a resting brachial-femoral systolic pressure gradient of 5 mm Hg or more or when papaverine injection (30 mg into the femoral artery) induces a drop in the brachial-femoral systolic pressure index of 15 percent or more.

A second limitation of the femorofemoral procedure is related to its lower patency rate when performed in a patient with superficial femoral artery occlusive disease. Unlike aortofemoral bypass, patency rates may be reduced by one half when the outflow is limited to the profunda femoris artery. A femorofemoral bypass may fail to relieve the patient's symptoms if the superficial femoral artery is occluded.

*Femorofemoral Bypass*

## OPERATIVE PROCEDURE

Femorofemoral bypass may be performed under general or regional anesthesia; local anesthesia may be used for a compromised patient. The common femoral arteries are exposed through bilateral groin incisions, and a suprapubic, subcutaneous tunnel is digitally developed (Fig. 84). The midline fascial attachments are pierced with the aid of an aortic clamp, and the graft is pulled through the tunnel without twists or kinks (Fig. 85). This creates the preferred inverted-C configuration, allowing long anastomoses to be constructed in an end-to-side fashion bilaterally. The anastomoses are continued onto the profunda femoris arteries in the form of profundaplasties if the superficial femoral artery is occluded. We prefer an 8-mm coated polyester or externally supported ePTFE graft.

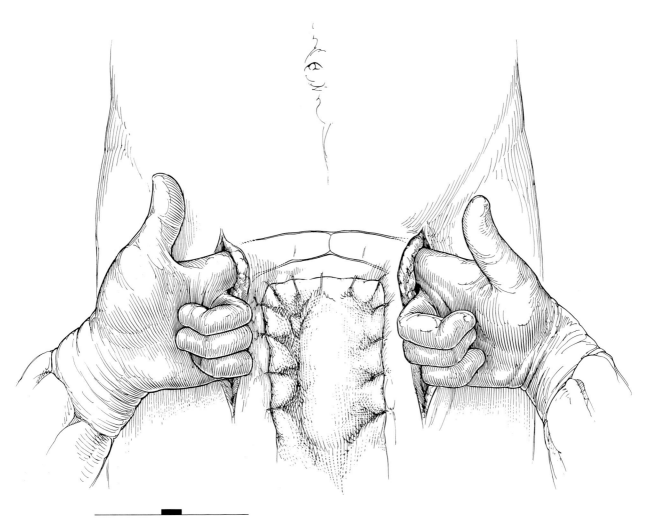

## Figure 84

The suprapubic tunnel is created digitally.

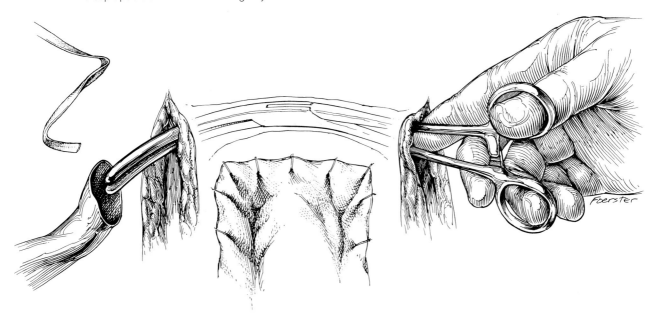

## Figure 85

The midline fascia is pierced with a long clamp, grasping a Penrose drain or an umbilical tape to facilitate delivery of the graft without kinks or twists.

## *Femorofemoral Bypass*

After heparin anticoagulation, the femoral anastomoses are constructed, preferably simultaneously with a two-team approach and employing 5-0 or 6-0 polypropylene suture in a running fashion (Fig. 86). Air is evacuated from the graft before removing the clamps, protamine is administered, and the wounds are closed in multiple layers.

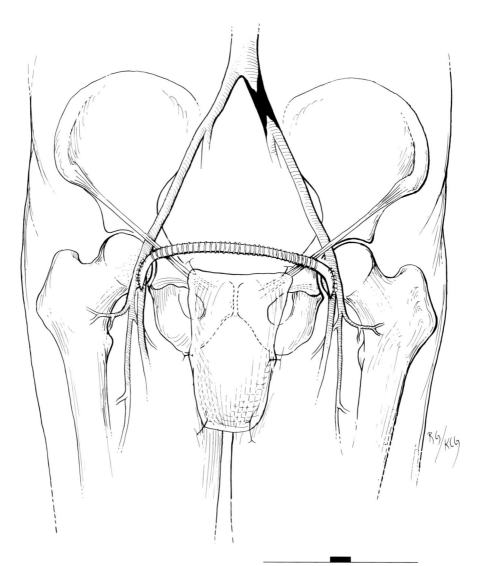

### Figure 86

Bilateral end-to-side anastomoses are constructed, each anastomosis being run onto the profunda femoris artery if the superficial femoral arteries are occluded.

# CHAPTER 14

# Axillofemoral Bypass

The axillofemoral bypass is an alternative approach used in the compromised patient with aortoiliac occlusive disease. The procedure also plays an important role in patients with aortic graft infections, providing a method with which to maintain lower extremity perfusion after excision of the aortic graft.

Axillofemoral bypass relies on a single axillary artery to provide perfusion to the lower extremities—a perfect scenario for a steal phenomenon when performed in the presence of an occult lesion in the donor subclavian system. Compromised with respect to long-term patency, axillofemoral reconstruction nevertheless avoids the morbidity associated with an abdominal operation and aortic clamping. Satisfactory long-term results may be achieved when outflow is ideal, and reoperation for acute axillofemoral graft thrombosis is frequently fruitful under local anesthesia alone. Axillobifemoral bypass is preferred to axillounifemoral bypass, because patency rates are higher when the outflow is directed to both lower extremities.

The axillobifemoral bypass should be envisioned as a standard femorofemoral bypass, attaching the axillary limb to the hood of the ipsilateral (i.e., donor side) anastomosis. In this manner, flow is maximized throughout the axillary limb, in contrast to the reduced flow produced in the distal ipsilateral segment when a bifurcated configuration is used.

*Axillofemoral Bypass*

# OPERATIVE PROCEDURE

General anesthesia is almost always necessary when performing an axillofemoral reconstruction. The donor upper extremity is abducted to 90° and placed on an arm board, affording the surgeon the option of standing on either side of the shoulder. The upper arm, shoulder, supraclavicular regions, ipsilateral chest, abdomen, and both groins are sterilely prepared and draped. A two-team approach is most efficient, with one surgeon performing the axillary anastomosis and the other the femorofemoral bypass.

An incision is made in the infraclavicular region, over the axillary artery. Whereas the standard incision for axillary artery exposure parallels the lower border of the clavicle, we prefer to place the incision at a 45° angle, running from a point just below the midpoint of the clavicle inferolaterally toward the lower border of the pectoralis major muscle (Fig. 87). This oblique incision directly overlies the pectoralis minor muscle and the axillary artery. The subcutaneous tissue is sharply divided, as is the pectoralis major muscle fascia. The underlying fibers of the pectoralis major muscle are bluntly separated and kept apart with the aid of a self-retaining retractor.

The deep fascia is then divided, exposing the triangular pectoralis muscle. The muscle assumes a tendinous appearance as it inserts on the coracoid process. Just as the division of the anterior scalene muscle provides access to the subclavian artery in the neck, the pectoralis minor muscle may be thought of as the gateway to the axillary artery. A finger is inserted beneath the uppermost portion of the muscle to assist in division with the electrocautery (Fig. 88). The pulsating axillary artery comes into view as the last fibers of the muscle are separated. The graft (usually an 8-mm ePTFE or coated polyester graft) is tunneled from the axillary wound, running deep to the pectoralis major muscle to reach the groin wound without the aid of a counterincision in all but the tallest of patients.

After heparin anticoagulation, the axillary artery and its branches are clamped (Fig. 89). Failure to control large inferior branches results in unexpected, brisk backbleeding from the arteriotomy. The anastomosis is placed just medial to the pectoralis minor muscle to avoid anastomotic disruption during vigorous abduction of the arm. The arteriotomy is made on the anteroinferior aspect of the axillary artery, avoiding injury to the posterior wall of the artery with the knife blade. An inadvertent incision in the back wall of the artery is possible with the No. 11 blade when the clamps cause the vessel to loop forward.

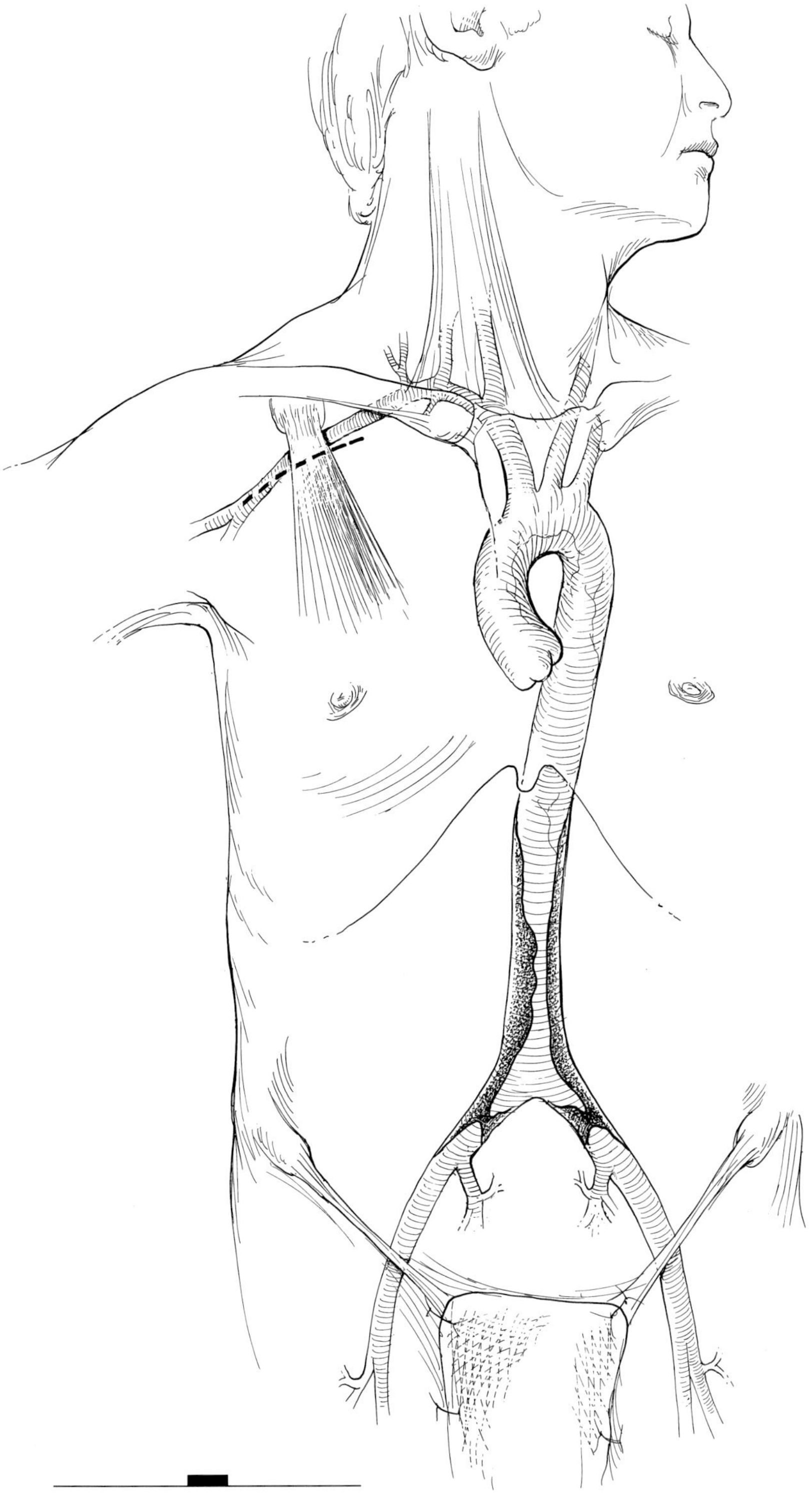

## Figure 87

The axillary artery is exposed through an oblique incision placed over the pectoralis minor muscle.

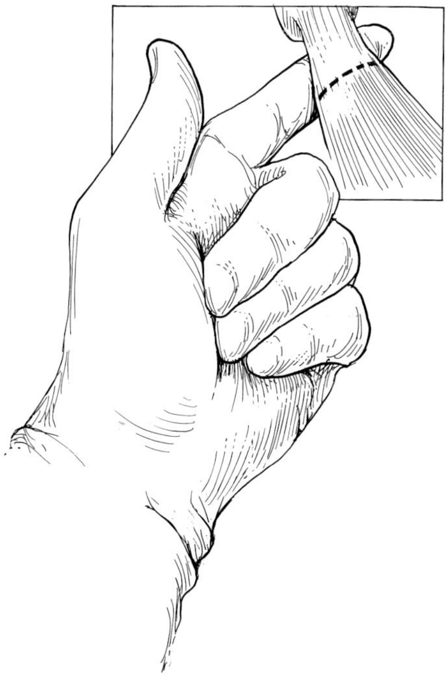

## Figure 88

The pectoralis minor muscle tendon is divided with the electrocautery, exposing the axillary artery running directly beneath the muscle.

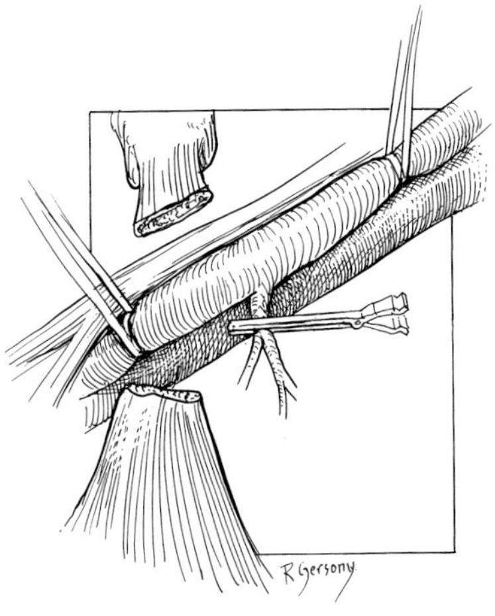


## Figure 89

The axillary artery is clamped, as are its large branches.

## Axillofemoral Bypass

A beveled anastomosis is constructed with 5-0 or 6-0 polypropylene suture (Fig. 90). The graft runs almost parallel to the artery and then exits the axilla beneath the pectoralis major muscle (Fig. 91). The axillary graft limb is anastomosed to the hood of the femorofemoral graft in the groin (Fig. 92), maximizing flow through the complete length of the axillofemoral graft limb. Gore-Tex suture is a good choice when anastomosing ePTFE grafts to one another, because suture-hole bleeding is sometimes diminished.

Air is flushed from the grafts before the outflow is opened, and the legs are sequentially released to decrease the hypotensive response. The adequacy of the reconstruction is confirmed with Doppler ultrasonography, duplex scanning, or intraoperative arteriography. The effect of heparin is reversed with protamine sulfate, and the wounds are closed in layers.

Late postoperative thrombosis of an axillofemoral graft may be easily treated under local anesthesia, exposing the graft through a small incision over the lateral tunnel. Alternatively, thrombolytic therapy may be employed, using a crossed two-catheter technique and accessing the graft along the lateral chest wall. The ease of revision of axillofemoral grafts accounts for a large difference between primary and secondary patency rates.

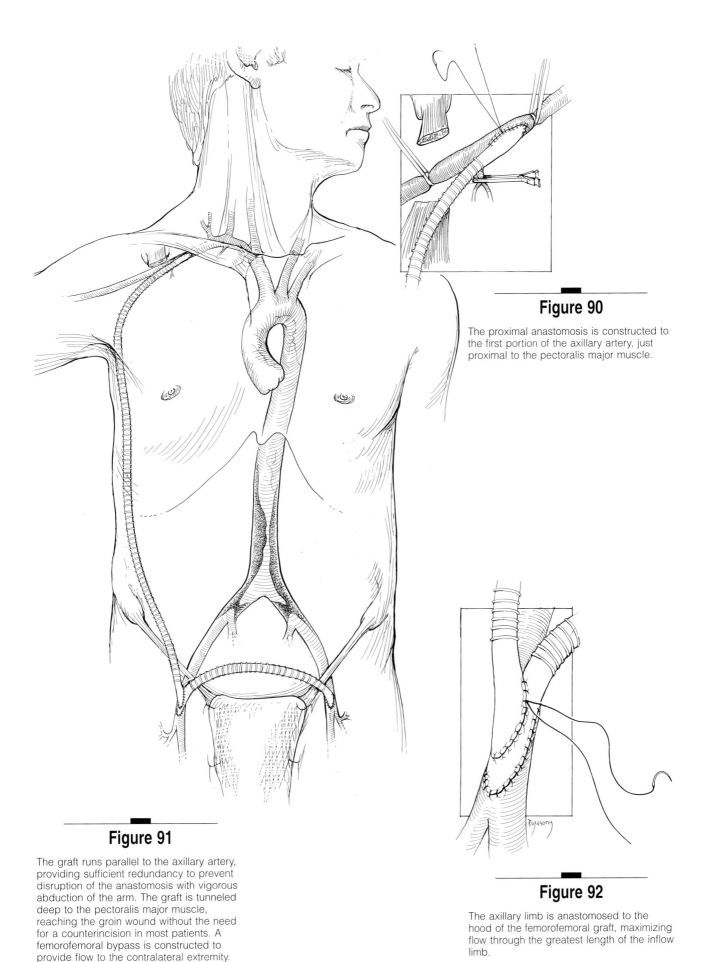

**Figure 90**

The proximal anastomosis is constructed to the first portion of the axillary artery, just proximal to the pectoralis major muscle.

**Figure 91**

The graft runs parallel to the axillary artery, providing sufficient redundancy to prevent disruption of the anastomosis with vigorous abduction of the arm. The graft is tunneled deep to the pectoralis major muscle, reaching the groin wound without the need for a counterincision in most patients. A femorofemoral bypass is constructed to provide flow to the contralateral extremity.

**Figure 92**

The axillary limb is anastomosed to the hood of the femorofemoral graft, maximizing flow through the greatest length of the inflow limb.

# ANEURYSM RESECTION

# CHAPTER 15

# Abdominal Aortic Aneurysm Resection

Abdominal aortic aneurysms are electively repaired to prevent rupture or, occasionally, distal embolization. Size is considered to be the primary correlate of rupture. Aortic aneurysms less than 5 cm in diameter are rarely associated with rupture, and resection is not necessary unless distal embolization has occurred. Aneurysms between 5 and 6 cm in diameter—and sometimes those between 4 and 5 cm—are repaired in healthy patients with a good longevity outlook. Larger aneurysms are associated with a progressively greater risk of rupture, and intervention is indicated in all but the most medically compromised patients.

Fortunately, more than 90 percent of abdominal aortic aneurysms begin below the level of the renal arteries. This feature allows the surgeon to approach most aneurysms transabdominally and still achieve adequate proximal control. Alternative methods of exposure can be used in selected clinical circumstances, but the midline transabdominal procedure is the most widely employed approach and is considered the standard against which all other methods must be compared. Nevertheless, as described in Chapter 17, the retroperitoneal approach offers some advantages in uncomplicated tube graft repairs. The retroperitoneal exposure has significant advantages in the settings of an inflammatory aneurysm, hostile abdomen, horseshoe kidney, and morbid obesity.

## OPERATIVE PROCEDURE

The patient is placed supine on the operating table, with wide preparation from the nipples to the mid-thigh level. We also include both legs to the ankle level in case a concurrent infrainguinal procedure becomes necessary. A plastic Steri-Drape aids in isolation of the groin from the sterile field. Mechanical retractors provide adequate exposure without multiple assistants. Otherwise, the second assistant stands to the cranial side of the surgeon, aiding in the retraction of the duodenum and small bowel (Fig. 93).

A radial arterial line and large-bore (16-gauge) peripheral intravenous line are employed. Frequently, a 14F introducer sheath is placed in an internal jugular or subclavian vein. A pulmonary artery catheter is used in cardiac-compromised patients. Alternatively, continuous transesophageal echocardiography may replace pulmonary arterial monitoring, with an increased sensitivity for early myocardial ischemia heralded by new wall motion abnormalities. An epidural catheter is used in many patients, because it lessens the need for deep general anesthesia and allows earlier extubation.

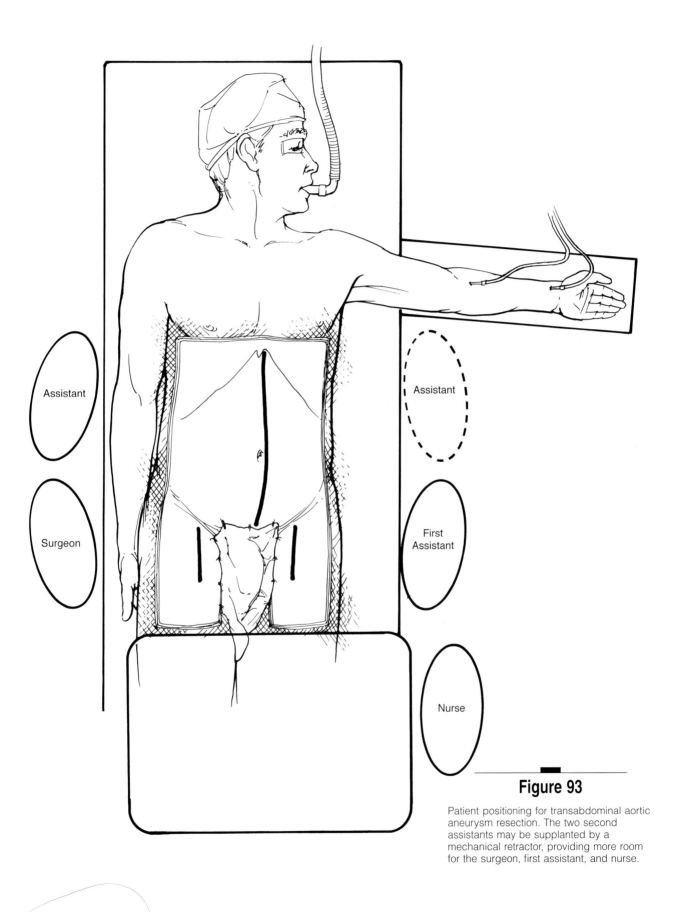

**Figure 93**

Patient positioning for transabdominal aortic aneurysm resection. The two second assistants may be supplanted by a mechanical retractor, providing more room for the surgeon, first assistant, and nurse.

## Abdominal Aortic Aneurysm Resection

The abdomen is opened through a long midline incision extending from the xiphoid to the pubis. After a thorough abdominal exploration, the duodenum and small bowel are mobilized to the right by incising the filmy attachments to the left of the duodenum. The duodenal mobilization is most easily accomplished by grasping the retroperitoneal tissues between two forceps, creating a small opening in the peritoneal layer with scissors, and inserting a finger beneath the tissue. The retroperitoneum is then incised with the electrocautery, repeating a similar maneuver and proceeding inferiorly to the level of the iliac arteries. The mobilization and retraction of the small bowel to the right displaces the thin, avascular midline tissues of the retroperitoneum in the same direction. The incision of the retroperitoneum is carried down over the right iliac artery to avoid the vessels within the sigmoid mesentery (Fig. 94).

The duodenum and small bowel are placed behind a large pad and retracted to the right with a fence retractor. Next, the tissue overlying the aorta is incised from the level of the left renal vein to the aortic bifurcation, clipping or ligating any traversing lymphatics and small vessels. The inferior mesenteric vein is identified and left undisturbed, keeping the retroperitoneal dissection to the right of the vein. Avulsion of the vein from the splenic or superior mesenteric vein is possible during retraction—an injury that may become evident only as the retractors are later removed. If injured, the inferior mesenteric vein can be ligated with impunity.

The surface of the aneurysm is cleared of tissue, keeping to the right of the inferior mesenteric artery (IMA) in preparation for an aortotomy that deliberately skirts the IMA orifice in case reimplantation of the vessel is deemed necessary. The IMA is controlled with a Potts double loop of Silastic, unless the artery is known to be chronically occluded.

Occasionally, high aneurysms may require medial division of the left renal vein to obtain adequate exposure for the proximal clamp (Fig. 95). This is well tolerated if the adrenal, gonadal, and ascending lumbar tributaries are left undisturbed and can serve as collateral outflow. Alternatively, a narrow renal vein retractor can be used (Fig. 96). In either case, care should be taken in upward retraction to avoid injury to a frequently atherosclerotic superior mesenteric artery (SMA). The SMA is found within the root of the small bowel mesentery as the vessel leaves the aorta to course over the duodenum, making it a prime target for injury from a forcefully placed retractor. The left gonadal and ascending lumbar veins may also be torn from vigorous cephalad retraction of the left renal vein or may be inadvertently incised during exposure of the aortic neck.

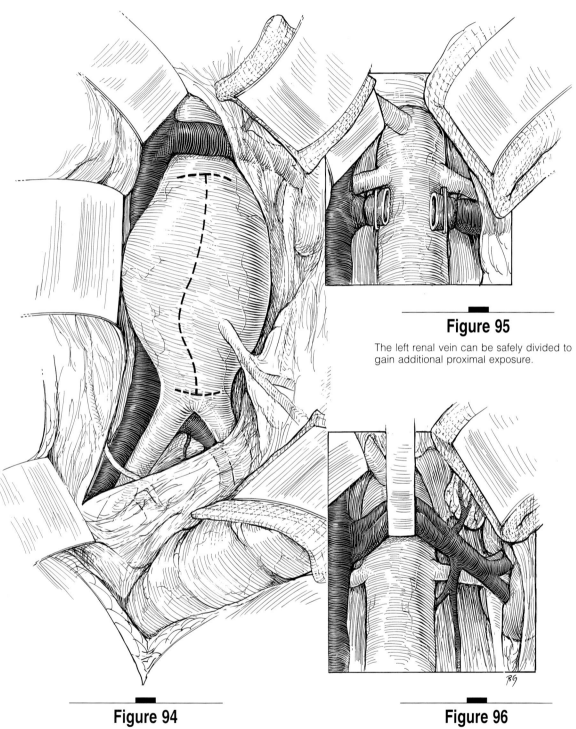

**Figure 95**

The left renal vein can be safely divided to gain additional proximal exposure.

**Figure 94**

The small bowel and duodenum are retracted to the right, placed behind a wide blade retractor. The retroperitoneum is incised to enter the plane just above the aortic adventitia. The incision extends from the renal vein to the right iliac artery, running along the avascular midline, which has been displaced to the right by retraction of the small intestine. The iliac arteries are not circumferentially dissected; only the anterior aspect of the vessels requires exposure for placement of the occluding clamps.

**Figure 96**

Alternatively, a narrow blade retractor may be positioned to draw the renal vein cephalad, exposing the pararenal aortic segment.

## *Abdominal Aortic Aneurysm Resection*

The aneurysm itself is not fully mobilized to avoid embolization of its friable contents to the legs, colon, or pelvis. Additional dissection is limited to the neck of the aneurysm just below the renal vein and the midportion of the common iliac arteries. There is no need to dissect circumferentially around the aorta or iliac vessels, but the anterior-most 270° must be exposed to safely apply the occluding clamps. A finger is carefully inserted to the side of the neck of the aneurysm (Fig. 97). A clamp can then be applied without dissection of the posterior aspect of the aorta.

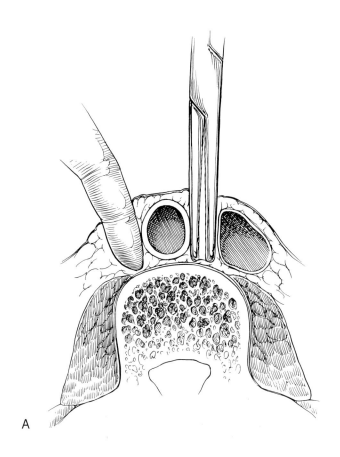

A

### Figure 97

Proximal control of the aortic neck is achieved with digital dissection along the sides of the aorta, just below the renal arteries. *A*, The bony vertebral bodies are palpated. *B*, Vertical pressure is applied as the jaws of the clamp firmly abut the bone. *C*, The clamp is closed, and inflow is occluded, achieving adequate proximal control without full circumferential dissection of the aorta.

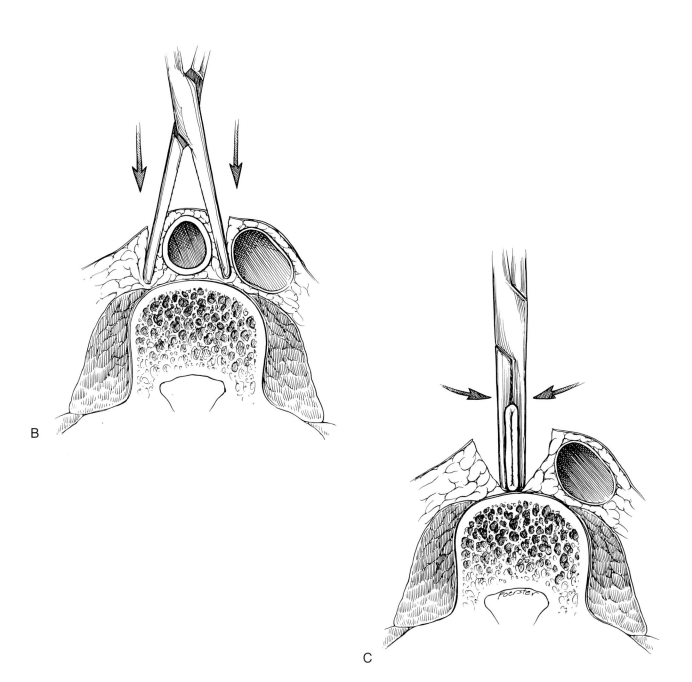

B

C

## Abdominal Aortic Aneurysm Resection

Supraceliac control of the aorta may be advantageous in certain patients, including those with pararenal involvement, inflammatory aneurysms, and ruptured aneurysms. In these cases, the aortic neck is left undisturbed, and attention is directed to the aorta as it exits from the diaphragmatic hiatus. The left lobe of the liver is mobilized to the right by complete division of its triangular ligament. The lesser omentum is divided perpendicularly (Fig. 98). The fibers of the crura of the diaphragm are spread digitally (Fig. 99) or, if time allows, sharply divided transversely to expose a sufficient length of supraceliac aorta for application of an occluding clamp (Fig. 100). Failure to unroof the crural fibers results in faulty application of the clamp, allowing it to slip off anteriorly.

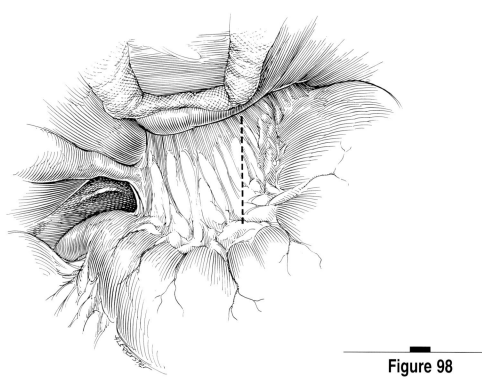

## Figure 98

When infrarenal aortic clamping is dangerous, a supraceliac position is useful. This situation arises in the case of a ruptured aortic aneurysm, an inflammatory aneurysm, or a pararenal aneurysm. The left lobe of the liver is mobilized and retracted to the right, with division of the triangular ligament. The lesser omentum is incised longitudinally.

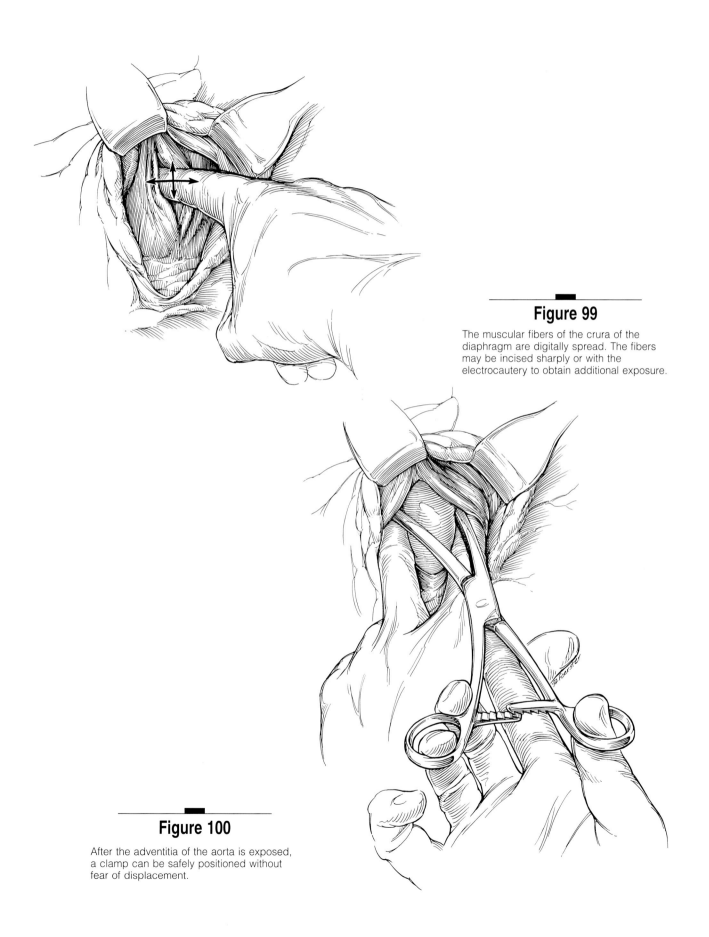

## Figure 99

The muscular fibers of the crura of the diaphragm are digitally spread. The fibers may be incised sharply or with the electrocautery to obtain additional exposure.

## Figure 100

After the adventitia of the aorta is exposed, a clamp can be safely positioned without fear of displacement.

## Abdominal Aortic Aneurysm Resection

Insertion of a tube graft is possible in a large percentage of patients undergoing abdominal aortic aneurysm repair. Heparin is administered before cross-clamping. The iliac vessels are clamped first, followed by the infrarenal aorta (Fig. 101). The aorta is opened longitudinally, "T'ing off" the aortotomy proximally and distally. The compacted thrombus within the aneurysm sac is digitally removed, and the lumen is flushed at the proximal and distal cuffs with saline solution or by momentary release of the clamps.

A Weitlaner retractor is placed within the lumen of the aneurysm to assist in the exposure of its interior. Lumbar vessels are oversewn with mattress sutures. Occasionally, an overlying portion of densely calcific aortic plaque needs to be removed to place the occluding sutures.

A vigorously backbleeding inferior mesenteric artery may be safely oversewn at this time, placing sutures from within the aneurysm sac to avoid occluding the proximal IMA branches. A low threshold should be maintained for reimplantation of the IMA. Relative indications for reimplantation include known SMA occlusive disease or the presence of a meandering mesenteric artery observed with arteriography. An IMA stump pressure below 40 mm Hg has been used to confirm the need for reimplantation, but the presence of a large, patent IMA with marginal backbleeding is usually sufficient reason to reimplant the vessel. This problem is more likely to arise if hypogastric flow is not preserved (see Chapter 16).

The proximal anastomosis is begun after control of the lumbar backbleeding. A graft is chosen with a diameter approximating the diameter of the aortic cuff, and the anastomosis is performed with 2-0 or 3-0 polypropylene suture (Fig. 102). The deep posterior bites serve to incorporate a double thickness of aortic wall with each pass. Upward traction on the suture creates a nice sewing ring if the aortic wall is pliable. Such a ring cannot be created in a very diseased and rigid aorta, for which a limited endarterectomy is sometimes necessary when the needle cannot penetrate the dense plaque.

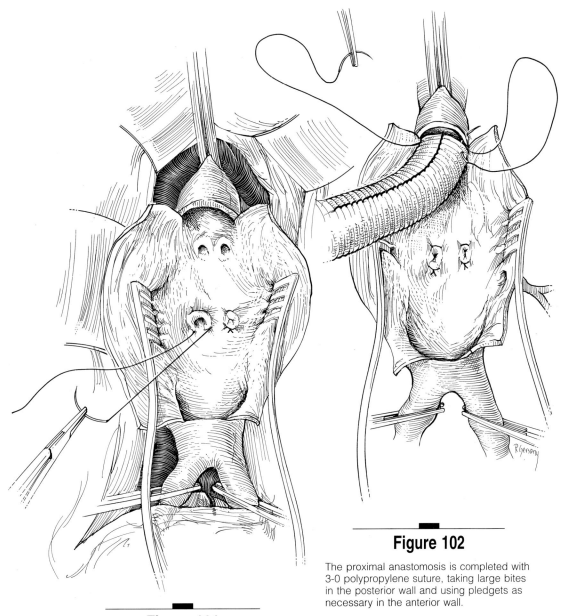

**Figure 101**

The aneurysm is opened, and the grumous thrombotic material is digitally removed. The proximal and distal necks are "T-ed" off, leaving the posterior wall intact. Lumbar backbleeding is controlled with mattress sutures placed at each orifice. When suture placement is impossible because of dense calcification, the plaque can be removed by local avulsion with a clamp. Inferior mesenteric backflow is assessed at this time. If the flow is brisk, the vessel is oversewn from within the aneurysm sac in a manner identical to that used for the lumbar arteries. If the mesenteric backbleeding is scant (and does not improve after restoration of aortic flow), the orifice should be excised for subsequent reimplantation onto the body of the graft.

**Figure 102**

The proximal anastomosis is completed with 3-0 polypropylene suture, taking large bites in the posterior wall and using pledgets as necessary in the anterior wall.

## *Abdominal Aortic Aneurysm Resection*

After completion of the proximal anastomosis, the clamp is moved to the midportion of the graft, and the anastomosis is inspected for significant leaks. Additional hemostatic sutures are placed as necessary, usually in a mattress configuration, with pledget sutures as needed. It is wise to briefly flush the graft again at this point to remove loose debris from the aortic cuff.

The distal anastomosis may be performed to the aortic bifurcation in a tube or straight configuration if three conditions are met. First, the iliac arteries must be nonaneurysmal, usually less than 2.5 cm in diameter. Second, there should be no significant iliac narrowing. Third, the aortic bifurcation should not be so severely calcified that, even with the aid of a localized endarterectomy, the anastomosis cannot be safely completed. If these conditions are met, a tube graft is appropriate, and the distal anastomosis is performed with 2-0 or 3-0 polypropylene suture in a manner similar to that of the proximal anastomosis (Fig. 103).

If it has been determined that reimplantation of the IMA is necessary, the orifice and a surrounding circle of aortic wall are excised from the aortic wall, and a limited endarterectomy is performed as needed. The IMA is implanted onto the anterolateral surface of the graft using 5-0 or 6-0 polypropylene suture (Fig. 104) and using a side-biting clamp on the body of the graft to allow lower extremity perfusion while the mesenteric anastomosis is completed.

Air is evacuated from the graft before release of the distal clamps by puncturing the graft with a 20-gauge needle. The iliac clamps are sequentially removed while closely monitoring the blood pressure as flow is returned to the legs. Transient hypotension is more common in aneurysmal disease than in occlusive disease as a result of fewer collaterals and a greater postocclusive hyperemic response. The feet are inspected, and distal pulses are palpated. If the IMA has been reimplanted, patency is confirmed with a Doppler probe.

Anticoagulation is reversed with protamine sulfate after adequate distal perfusion has been ensured. Hemostasis is achieved, and closing the retroperitoneum and aneurysm sac with a single layer of running suture covers the graft and anastomoses. Mobilized omentum may be used if the aneurysm is too small to completely cover the graft. The midline fascia and skin are then closed in standard fashion.

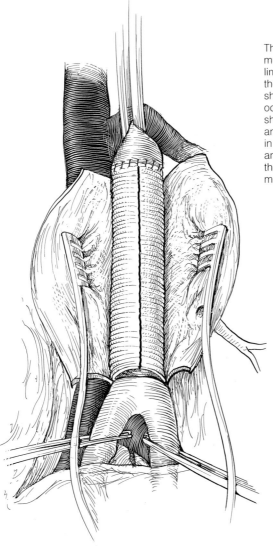

## Figure 103

The extent of calcium deposition usually is much greater distally than proximally. A limited endarterectomy is feasible to allow the placement of sutures, but the surgeon should be careful to prevent a flap from occluding the iliac outflow. A low threshold should be maintained for abandoning the anastomosis at the aortic bifurcation, acting in favor of a bifurcated graft configuration. If anastomosis to the bifurcation is possible, the distal anastomosis is completed in a manner analogous to that used proximally.

## Figure 104

A large inferior mesenteric artery with minimal backbleeding should be reimplanted onto the body of the graft. An endarterectomy of the proximal artery is usually necessary, everting the vessel to follow the plaque to a suitable end point. The anastomosis is performed with 5-0 or 6-0 polypropylene suture. A side-biting aortic clamp can be used to allow flow through the graft during reimplantation of the artery.

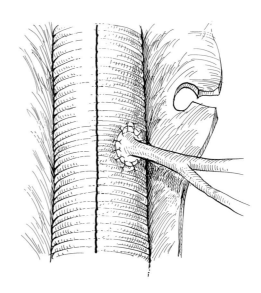

# CHAPTER 16

# Resection of Aortic Aneurysms Involving the Iliac Arteries

When aortic aneurysmal disease extends to involve the iliac arteries, the operative procedure and exposure become somewhat more complex. Iliac aneurysms should be resected in concert with the aortic aneurysm repair when their diameter is greater than 2.5 cm, but the life expectancy of the patient also should be taken into account.

The goals of the procedure are to exclude the aortic and iliac aneurysms and to restore flow to the lower extremities and pelvic circulation. Fortunately, most common iliac artery aneurysms end at the bifurcation into the hypogastric and external iliac arteries. In this circumstance, the prototypic procedure is an end-to-end reconstruction to the common iliac artery terminus.

Two disease processes may require modification of the operative plan: external iliac stenotic disease and hypogastric aneurysms. Significant occlusive disease of the external iliac arteries dictates a bypass to the femoral artery using groin incisions. In many cases, the distal external iliac artery is healthy just before its exit from beneath the inguinal ligament, and a groin incision can be avoided. In this case, the distal common iliac artery may be ligated or oversewn to provide retrograde perfusion of the hypogastric arteries from distal anastomotic sites.

Hypogastric artery aneurysms represent a more difficult challenge, primarily because of the difficulties of operative exposure and the inability to restore pelvic circulation. When small, a hypogastric aneurysm may be excluded from the reconstruction, with proximal ligation performed at the hypogastric origin. When large, however, the aneurysm must be opened and the outflow branches individually oversewn by the technique of endoaneurysmorrhaphy. Hypogastric aneurysms usually reside deep in the pelvis, making this procedure technically difficult and threatening increased blood loss and, when performed bilaterally, the attendant risk of ischemia to the buttocks, colon, and spinal cord.

## OPERATIVE PROCEDURE

The aorta is exposed in the standard fashion, but a more caudal incision of the retroperitoneum is necessary to expose the origins of the external iliac and hypogastric arteries (Fig. 105). Whereas the distal right iliac system is easily exposed with continua-

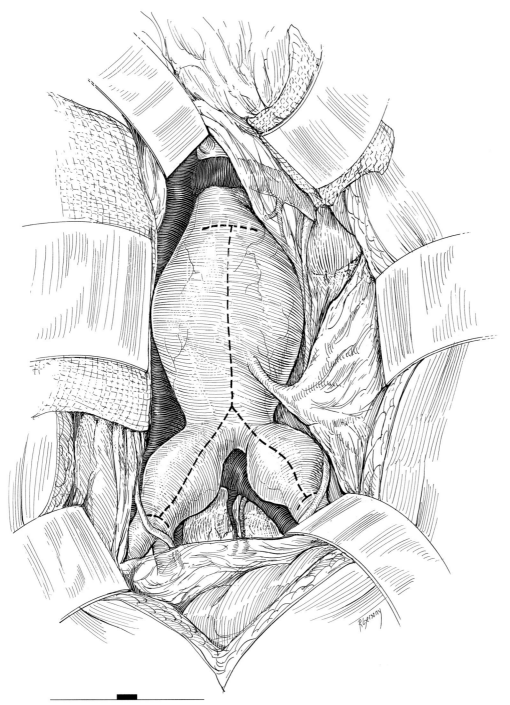

**Figure 105**

A more extensive exposure is required for
aortoiliac aneurysms than is necessary
when the process is confined to the
abdominal aorta. The common iliac arteries
are exposed to their bifurcations, with
extension of the retroperitoneal incision
toward the right and retraction of the
sigmoid colon and the inferior mesenteric
vessels to the left.

## Resection of Aortic Aneurysms Involving the Iliac Arteries

tion of the retroperitoneal incision, the left external iliac artery is better exposed through a separate incision lateral to the sigmoid colon (Fig. 106). The external iliac and hypogastric arteries should be separately controlled when iliac aneurysms extend to the bifurcation (Fig. 107), taking care to avoid injury to adherent iliac veins or ureters during the circumferential dissection of these vessels.

The body (i.e., common stem) of the bifurcated graft should be cut to a short length, usually 3 to 5 cm. Minimizing this length allows easier thrombectomy through the graft limbs, which is useful in the infrequent event of bilateral graft limb thrombosis. A long graft body encourages kinking of the graft limbs at the bifurcation. The proximal aortic anastomosis is performed in an essentially identical manner to that described earlier, but the surgeon must be creative in designing the configuration of the distal anastomoses.

Ideally, the iliac graft limbs may be sewn directly to the common iliac bifurcation in an end-to-end fashion (Fig. 108). After the proximal anastomosis is constructed in the usual fashion, releasing the aortic clamp and individually clamping the iliac graft limbs, the distal anastomoses are performed to the iliac bifurcations by transecting the distal common iliac artery or by constructing the suture line from within the iliac aneurysm. In this fashion, normal, antegrade perfusion of the hypogastric arteries is maintained, with little risk of pelvic ischemia.

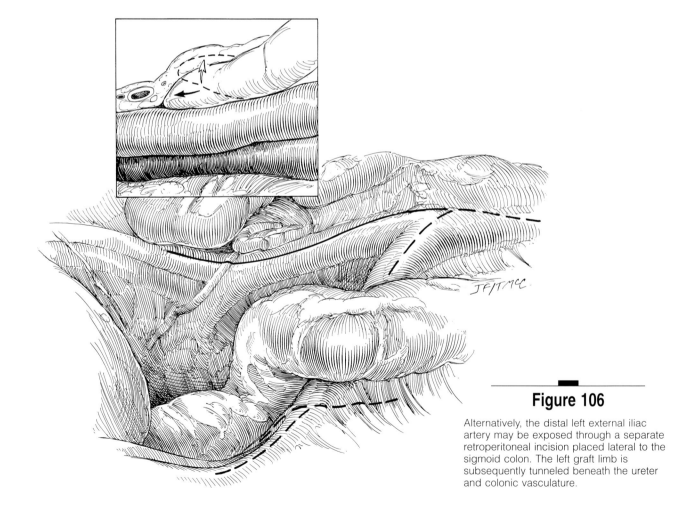

### Figure 106

Alternatively, the distal left external iliac artery may be exposed through a separate retroperitoneal incision placed lateral to the sigmoid colon. The left graft limb is subsequently tunneled beneath the ureter and colonic vasculature.

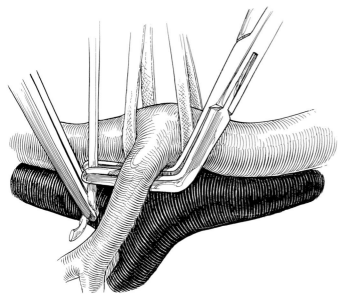

## Figure 107

The distal common iliac and proximal external iliac arteries are separately controlled, pulling up on the vessel tapes to gain hypogastric control.

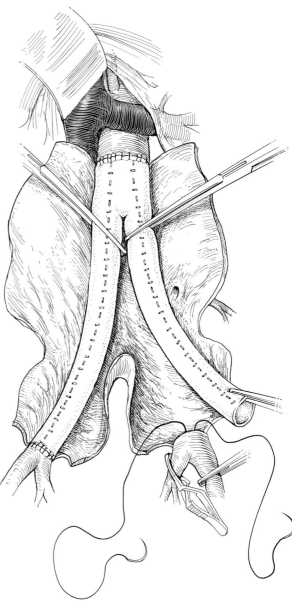

## Figure 108

The body of the graft is kept relatively short but with long limbs to prevent kinking and facilitate thrombectomy. The proximal anastomosis is completed in the usual fashion, sewing the posterior row from within the aneurysm sac. The distal anastomosis may be completed to the transected distal common iliac artery using 4-0 or 5-0 suture. Alternatively, the distal anastomosis can be completed from within the iliac aneurysm sac when the aneurysm is large, in a manner analogous to that used for the proximal anastomosis. This technique is most useful when the aneurysm extends to the iliac bifurcation.

## Resection of Aortic Aneurysms Involving the Iliac Arteries

Alternatively, the iliac graft limb may be anastomosed to the side of the distal external iliac artery with ligation or oversewing of the distal common iliac vessel (Fig. 109). This option is feasible only when the iliac aneurysm terminates with a cuff of relatively normal sized iliac vessel proximal to the bifurcation.

The remainder of the procedure is similar to that of tube graft aortic reconstruction. The aneurysm is closed over the graft to prevent adherence of the bowel to the prosthetic material. Closure of the retroperitoneal layer is necessary to cover the graft limbs when the iliac aneurysms themselves are not large enough to close over the graft. The abdominal wound is then closed using standard techniques.

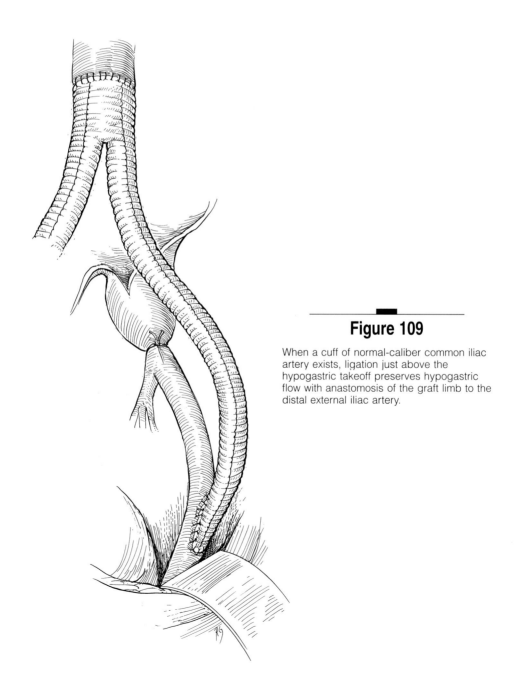

### Figure 109

When a cuff of normal-caliber common iliac artery exists, ligation just above the hypogastric takeoff preserves hypogastric flow with anastomosis of the graft limb to the distal external iliac artery.

# CHAPTER 17

# *Retroperitoneal Approach to Abdominal Aortic Aneurysms*

Traditionally, abdominal aortic aneurysm repair has been performed transperitoneally through a long midline incision. As an alternative approach, the retroperitoneal exposure offers advantages for specific subgroups of patients. In patients with pulmonary insufficiency, previous abdominal surgical procedures, inflammatory aneurysms, horseshoe kidney, or morbid obesity, abdominal aortic aneurysms may be best repaired through this approach.

Advantages of the retroperitoneal approach include the ability to easily expose the aorta at or above the level of the renal arteries. A retroperitoneal approach appears to cause less morbidity with regard to the duration of intestinal ileus and pulmonary complications, although the use of epidural catheters has closed this gap. A distinct disadvantage of the retroperitoneal approach is the inability to easily access the right iliac vessels. The right femoral artery also is more difficult to expose with the patient tilted in a full lateral decubitus position. Moreover, in certain patients, the tunnel between the retroperitoneal space and the right groin may be difficult to create and fraught with the risk of venous or ureteral injuries. For these reasons, the retroperitoneal approach is best applied in tube graft repairs of abdominal aortic aneurysms.

**Retroperitoneal Approach to Abdominal Aortic Aneurysms**

## OPERATIVE PROCEDURE

The patient is placed in a lateral decubitus position, with the left side of the body elevated 45° to 90° (Fig. 110). The legs and pelvis remain as flat as possible to facilitate groin exposure. The left arm is elevated over the chest and secured with a padded restraint.

A transverse flank incision is made, beginning at the tip of the 12th rib and continuing toward the umbilicus. Dissection is carried down through the muscular layers of the abdomen, incising the anterior rectus sheath and the rectus muscle itself but leaving the posterior rectus sheath and adherent peritoneum intact. The retroperitoneal space is entered laterally after identifying the proper plane of dissection by the yellow fat overlying the psoas muscle.

After the retroperitoneal space has been entered, care is taken to proceed more anteriorly, in front of the psoas muscle. To enlarge the exposure, the peritoneal sac is swept off the anterior and lateral aspects of the abdominal wall using blunt dissection. At this point, the posterior rectus sheath is carefully incised, leaving the underlying peritoneum intact, and the abdominal contents can be swept medially along with the ureter. Alternatively, the ureter can be left in its normal position, and the inferior mesenteric artery can be ligated or left intact (Fig. 111).

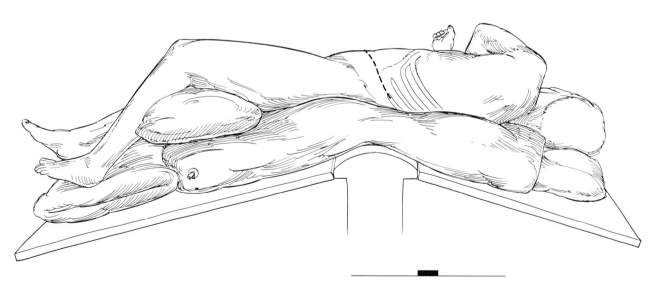

**Figure 110**

The patient is positioned in a lateral decubitus position with the chest at 45° to 90° and the pelvis almost level. The operating table is flexed to open the space between the costal margin and the pelvic brim.

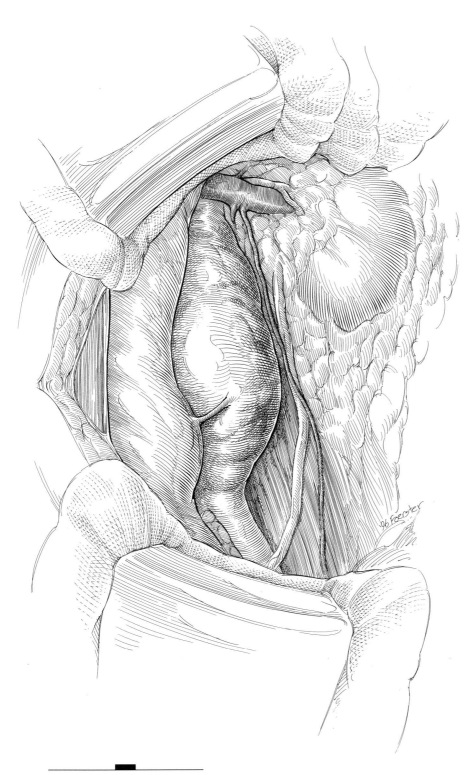

**Figure 111**

Exposure of the aneurysm, keeping the left
kidney in situ and reflecting the peritoneal
sac medially.

## Retroperitoneal Approach to Abdominal Aortic Aneurysms

The two options for aortic exposure using the retroperitoneal approach differ in the management of the left kidney. The kidney may be left in situ and the dissection plane developed anterior to Gerota's fascia. Alternatively, dissection can proceed posterior to the kidney, dividing the ascending lumbar vein and elevating the organ anteromedially along with the peritoneal contents (Fig. 112). The major difference between the two approaches is the position of the left renal vein. The renal vein lies in its normal position, overlying the aorta, when the kidney is left in situ. This approach is appropriate for aneurysms beginning below the renal arteries. Elevation of the kidney provides higher exposure of the abdominal aorta, with proximal aortic exposure limited only by the ability to retract the flank incision. The latter approach is ideal for juxtarenal or pararenal aneurysms, provided that the left renal vein is not retroaortic.

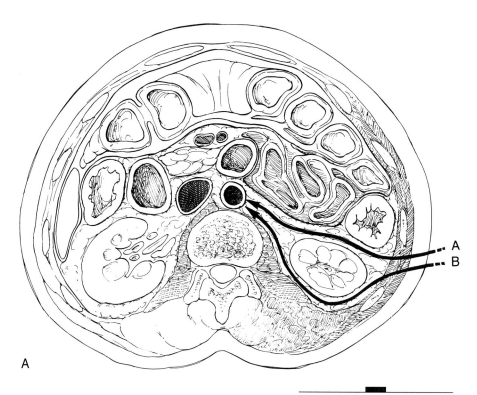

A

## Figure 112

Two approaches into the retroperitoneal structures. *A*, The first is anterior to the kidney and adrenal gland. *B*, The second is behind these organs, mobilizing them forward.

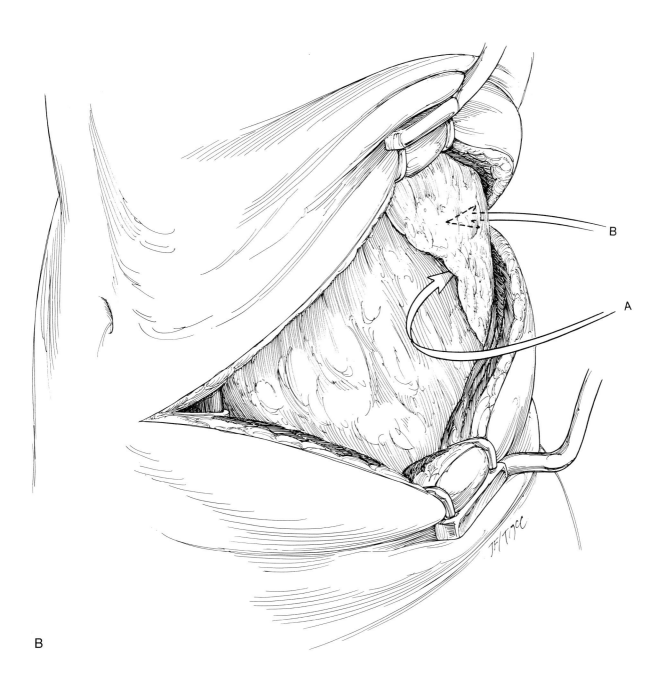

B

## *Retroperitoneal Approach to Abdominal Aortic Aneurysms*

Dissection is begun at the aortic neck, just below the level of the renal vein, when the kidney is not reflected anteriorly. In contrast to the transabdominal approach, in which the anterior and lateral aspects of proximal aortic neck are dissected free of surrounding tissue, in the retroperitoneal approach, the proximal aortic neck is cleared of tissue on its anterior, left lateral, and posterior aspects. An occluding aortic clamp is easily inserted from the left lateral position (Fig. 113). It is unnecessary to completely expose the right lateral aspect of the proximal aortic neck, except in the unusual circumstance when the aorta must be transected completely for the proximal anastomosis.

Exposure of the left iliac system is facilitated by the retroperitoneal approach, which permits good visualization of the iliac system to the most distal aspect of the external iliac artery. The left common iliac artery is easily prepared for clamping. Although exposure of the right common iliac artery is fairly straightforward in many cases, adequate exposure of this vessel may sometimes be arduous, and balloon catheter control is sometimes safer (Fig. 114). The proximal anastomosis then proceeds in a manner analogous to that with the standard, transabdominal approach. The distal anastomosis is completed in a similar fashion, removing the right iliac occlusion catheter just before placement of the last few sutures.

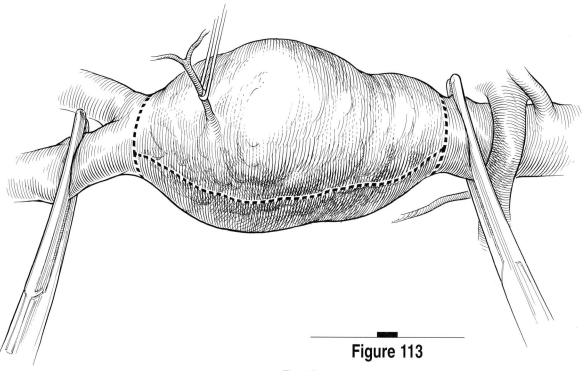

### Figure 113

The inferior mesenteric artery is occluded with a vessel loop, and the left iliac artery is clamped, as is the infrarenal aorta. The right iliac artery is left undissected and unclamped and is instead controlled with a balloon-occluding catheter.

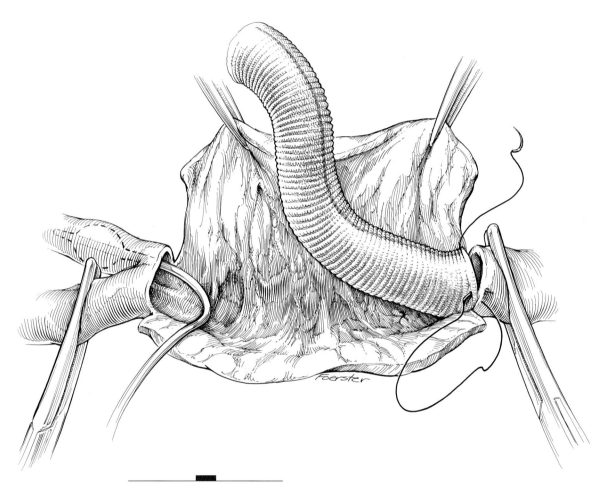

## Figure 114

A balloon-occluding catheter is positioned in the right common iliac artery. The proximal anastomosis is completed with 3-0 polypropylene suture in a manner identical to that employed in the standard, transabdominal approach.

## *Retroperitoneal Approach to Abdominal Aortic Aneurysms*

In some cases, the iliac orifices are not closely juxtaposed as they exit from the aneurysm sac. The orifices instead may have been moved far apart by dilatation of the bridging aneurysmal tissue between them. In these cases, it may be reasonable to use a bifurcated graft (Fig. 115), with the right iliac occluding balloon removed just before completion of the anastomosis.

Occasionally, the balloon catheter does not completely prevent backflow from the iliac artery, usually because the balloon has been placed too far into the iliac artery, beyond the hypogastric orifice. In other instances, continued backbleeding occurs because a markedly irregular atherosclerotic surface of the iliac artery thwarts complete occlusion by the surface of the balloon. In these cases, the operator can thread the balloon catheter through the graft, performing the distal anastomoses first to minimize the period of iliac backbleeding (Fig. 116). Thereafter, the balloon is removed, a clamp is placed on the midportion of the aortic graft, and the proximal anastomosis is performed.

After the anastomoses have been completed, the aneurysm sac is closed over the graft (Fig. 117). The peritoneal sac is returned to its normal position. The flank incision is closed using continuous absorbable suture for each muscular layer and clips for the skin.

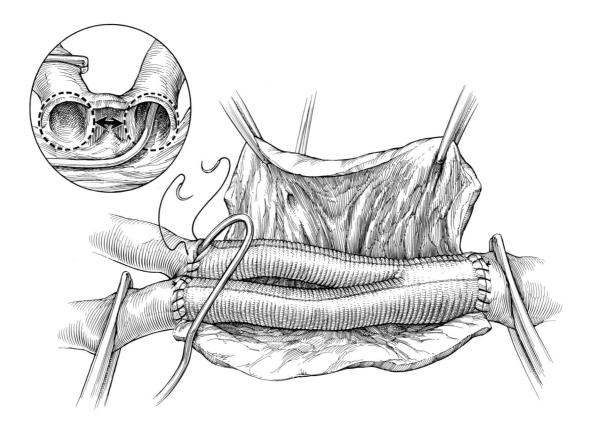

## Figure 115

Aneurysmal dilatation at the aortic bifurcation may expand the space between the iliac orifices *(inset)*. In this case, a bifurcated graft is appropriate, sewing each limb to the proximal common iliac vessels.

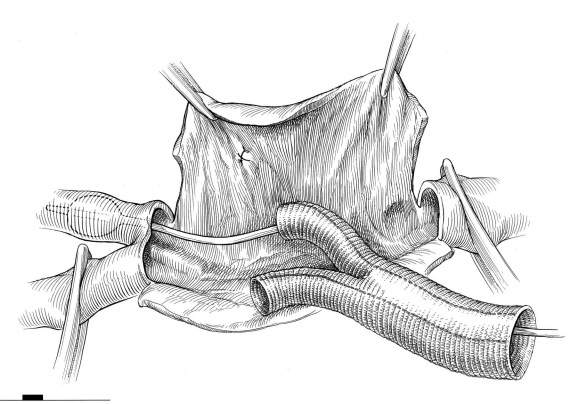

**Figure 116**

When the balloon catheter fails to
completely arrest iliac backbleeding, it is
best to complete the distal anastomoses
first. The balloon catheter is threaded
through the graft, and the iliac anastomoses
are performed. Thereafter, the balloon is
removed, a clamp is placed on the body of
the graft, and the proximal anaston
completed.

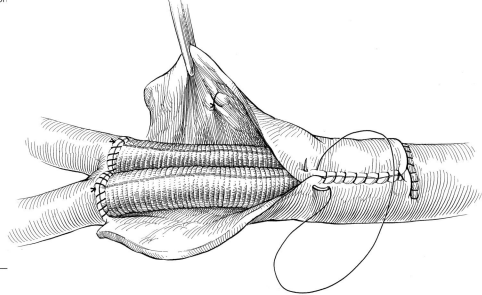

**Figure 117**

The aneurysm sac is closed over the graft
after completion of the anastomoses.

# CHAPTER 18

# *Thoracoabdominal Aneurysm Repair*

The repair of a thoracoabdominal aneurysm is perhaps one of the most technically demanding tasks in peripheral vascular surgery. The technical maneuvers in this procedure are arduous, and each maneuver must be performed quickly and efficiently to prevent ischemic injury to the kidneys and spinal cord. The hemodynamic, hematologic, and metabolic derangements that may occur during the performance of a thoracoabdominal aneurysm repair are reflected in its relatively high morbidity and mortality rates. Nevertheless, the technical innovations by such pioneers as E. Stanley Crawford, particularly his endoluminal "island inclusion" anastomotic technique for visceral artery orifices, have greatly reduced the morbidity of the procedure. Moreover, progress in the areas of anesthesia, spinal cord protective measures, intraoperative autotransfusion, and postoperative critical care have acted in concert with technical innovations to decrease the risk of thoracoabdominal aneurysm resection.

The morbidity and mortality of thoracoabdominal aneurysm repair correlates with the anatomic extent of disease. Dr. Crawford devised four categories of thoracoabdominal aneurysms. Type 1 thoracoabdominal aneurysms begin just beyond the left subclavian artery and terminate just above the level of the renal arteries. Type 2 aneurysms also begin just distal to the left of the subclavian artery, but they terminate at the aortic bifurcation, involving the aorta at the level of the visceral vessels. Type 3 aneurysms begin at the level of the mid-descending thoracic aorta and end, like type 2 aneurysms, at the aortic bifurcation. Type 4 aneurysms begin at the level of the diaphragm and terminate at the aortic bifurcation. The type 2 thoracoabdominal aneurysm is the most common variety and is also associated with the highest risk of complications, such as postoperative paraplegia.

## OPERATIVE PROCEDURE

After placement of large-bore venous access cannulas, anesthesia is induced. In high-risk cases, cerebrospinal fluid is drained perioperatively to decrease the risk of spinal cord ischemia. The catheter is placed in the L4-L5 vertebral space, and cerebrospinal fluid is drained by gravity to keep the spinal fluid pressure below 10 mm Hg. Drainage is continued for as long as 3 days after the operation. A radial artery line is placed on the right side in case clamping of the left subclavian artery becomes necessary. A double-lumen endotracheal tube is used for selective collapse of the left lung.

An autotransfusion device is used to collect and reinfuse blood shed during the operation. Many centers use partial left-heart bypass, cannulating the left inferior pulmonary vein and the femoral artery. A Bio-Medicus centrifugal pump is used to shunt

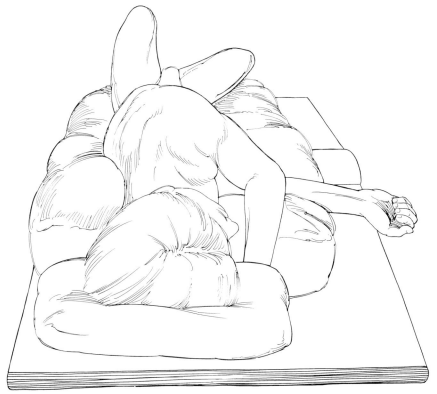

**Figure 118**

Patient positioning for resection of a thoracoabdominal aneurysm. The upper torso is placed in a full lateral position, and the pelvis is tilted at 30° to provide access to the groins. The use of a beanbag maintains patient positioning.

blood from the left atrium to one of the femoral arteries during the period of aortic cross-clamping. The use of a left-heart bypass minimizes the duration of visceral ischemia by allowing retrograde perfusion of the aorta during performance of the proximal anastomosis and permits selective perfusion of the renal, superior mesenteric, and celiac vessels through coronary perfusion cannulas during visceral reimplantation.

The patient is positioned in the right lateral decubitus position. A beanbag is used to keep the chest at 90° and the left hip at 45° to the plane of the operating table (Fig. 118). The left thoracoabdominal incision is made through the fifth, sixth, seventh, or eighth intercostal space, depending on the extent of proximal aortic involvement. A rib may be resected to facilitate wide exposure. In the past, the abdominal portion of the incision commonly was a midline laparotomy extending to the xiphoid process, connecting with the thoracic portion of the incision. In a newer approach, a laterally placed incision is used, continuing the chest incision in a linear fashion toward the umbilicus. The more laterally placed incision avoids the triangular area of skin and muscle necrosis that frequently developed at the junction of the midline abdominal and thoracic components of the older approach.

*Thoracoabdominal Aneurysm Repair*

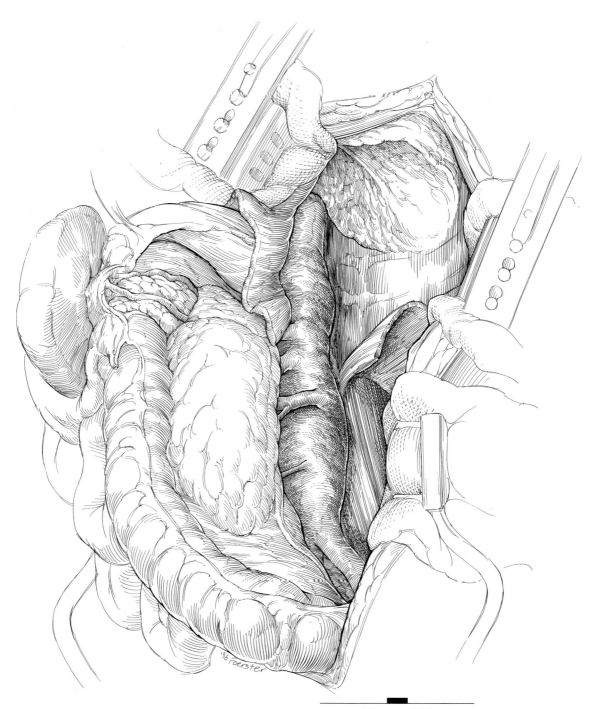

## Figure 119

The transperitoneal approach to exposure of
a thoracoabdominal aneurysm, using medial
visceral rotation. The left kidney has been
elevated anteromedially, and the ureter has
been retracted to the right along with the
peritoneal contents. The risk of splenic
injury and fluid loss from the exposed
viscera is greater with the transperitoneal
approach, but access to the right iliac
system is better than a thoraco-
retroperitoneal exposure.

The surgeon has two choices for exposing the abdominal portion of a thoracoabdominal aneurysm repair. In the first approach, the thoracic incision is connected with a midline abdominal incision. The peritoneal cavity is entered, and a medial visceral rotation is performed, elevating the left kidney out of the retroperitoneal space (Fig. 119). The diaphragm is split radially to the aortic hiatus (Fig. 120). Marking sutures can be placed at this time to facilitate more accurate reapproximation of the diaphragm during closure.

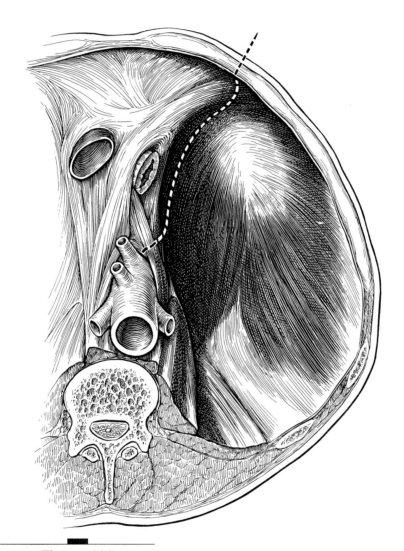

## Figure 120

The diaphragm is incised radially toward the aortic hiatus when using the transperitoneal approach.

## *Thoracoabdominal Aneurysm Repair*

The second approach to the abdominal portion of a thoracoabdominal aneurysm repair involves a "thoraco-retroperitoneal" exposure. The peritoneal cavity is not entered; rather, the plane of dissection is kept within the retroperitoneal space, reflecting the left kidney anteriorly. The diaphragm is incised circumferentially (Fig. 121), leaving an adequate rim for reattachment. Figure 122 illustrates the exposure of a type 1 thoracoabdominal aneurysm using a transperitoneal approach. Exposure of the aneurysm proceeds along the posterolateral aspect of the aneurysm. In all cases, care must be taken to protect the left renal artery, which is easily injured as it courses toward the elevated left kidney. Figure 123 depicts the course of the left renal artery after elevation of the left kidney in a type 3 thoracoabdominal aneurysm. Access to the right iliac system is more difficult when using a thoraco-retroperitoneal approach, but fluid shifts and the risk of injury to the spleen are lessened.

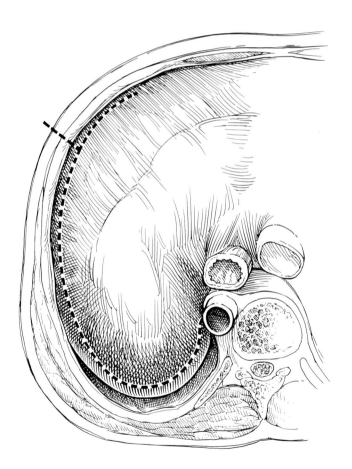

## Figure 121

The diaphragm is incised circumferentially when using a thoraco-retroperitoneal exposure, leaving an ample rim for subsequent reattachment. The circumferential technique is associated with improved postoperative function, because it minimizes damage to the phrenic nerve branches.

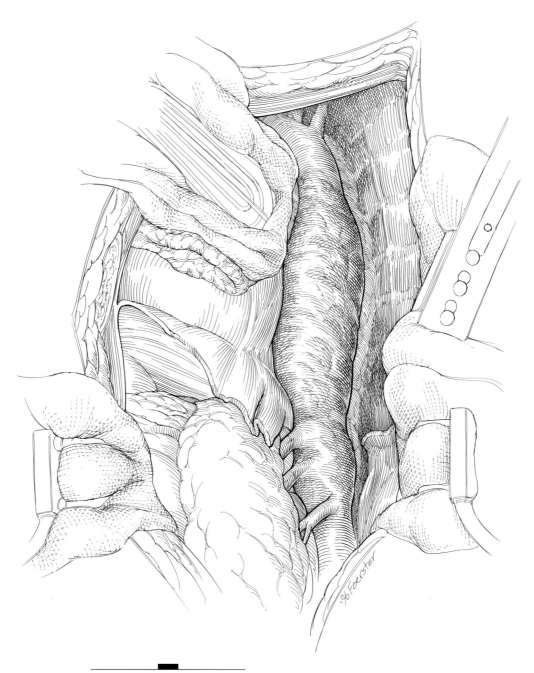

**Figure 122**

Transperitoneal exposure of a type 1
thoracoabdominal aneurysm.

## Thoracoabdominal Aneurysm Repair

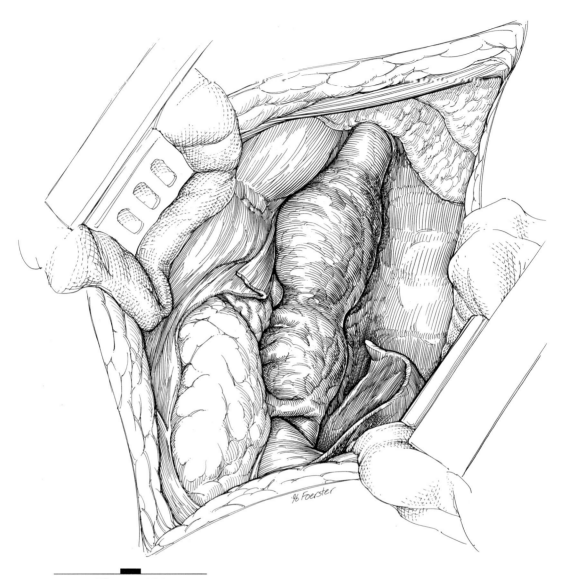

## Figure 123

The exposure of a type 3 thoracoabdominal aneurysm, illustrating the position of the left renal artery, which may be inadvertently injured as it courses over the dilated aorta.

After the proximal and distal extents of the aneurysm have been well exposed, the origins of the celiac, superior mesenteric, and left renal vessels are identified and dissected free of surrounding tissue (Fig. 124). Often, the visceral and renal vessels are obscured by the aneurysm or surrounding inflammatory change, and formal exposure of the vessels is unwise. The inferior mesenteric artery may be ligated and divided at this point if additional retraction of the peritoneal sac and exposure of the right iliac system are necessary. The large ascending lumbar vein commonly empties into the left renal vein. This vein must be ligated to prevent troublesome venous bleeding.

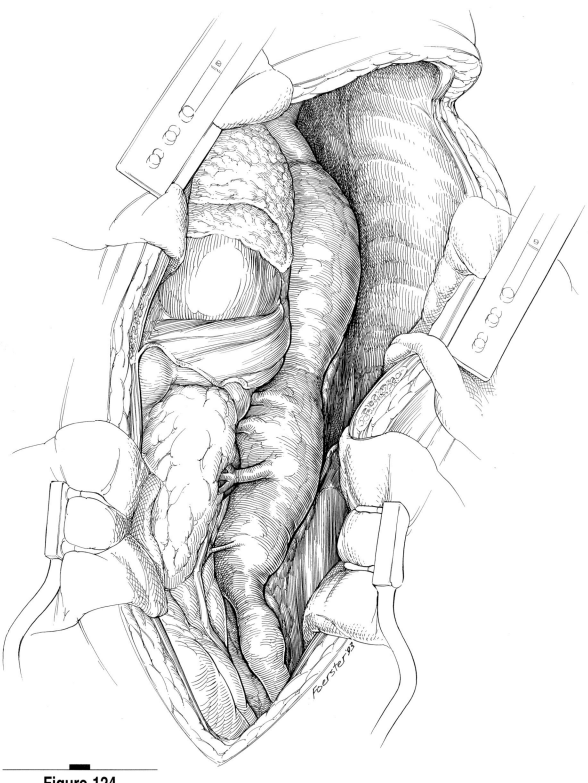

**Figure 124**

Exposure of the origins of the visceral
vessels in a type 2 thoracoabdominal aortic
aneurysm involving the left iliac system.

## Thoracoabdominal Aneurysm Repair

Figure 125 illustrates this maneuver in a type 4 thoracoabdominal aneurysm. The aneurysm has been exposed, as have the visceral vessels and left iliac artery. To avoid the difficulties associated with exposure of the right iliac artery, preparation should be made for the use of an occluding balloon cannula.

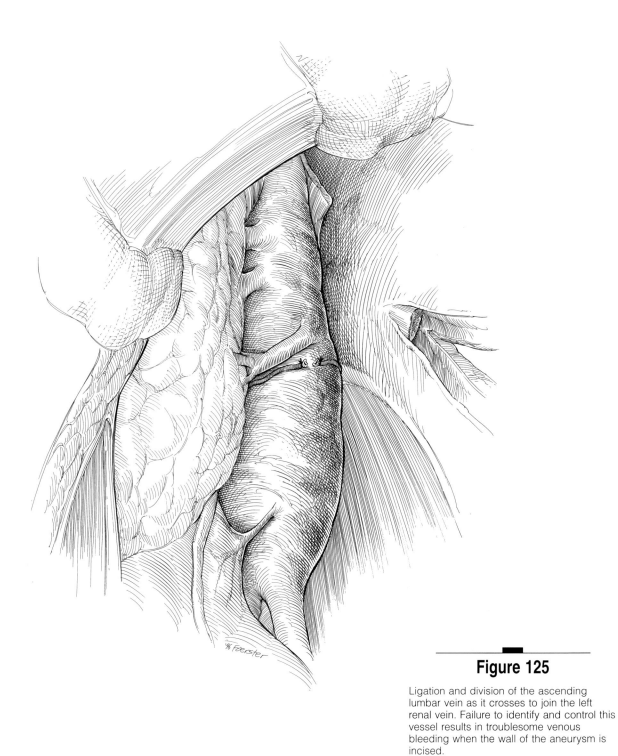

**Figure 125**

Ligation and division of the ascending lumbar vein as it crosses to join the left renal vein. Failure to identify and control this vessel results in troublesome venous bleeding when the wall of the aneurysm is incised.

Heparin may or may not be administered during the procedure, but when a Bio-Medicus pump is employed, moderate-dose heparin (5000 to 10,000 units as a bolus) is used. The distal clamps are placed, followed by the proximal aortic clamp (Fig. 126). The aorta is opened along a posterolateral line while care is taken to remain posterior to the left renal orifice. The proximal and distal cuffs are "T-ed." The right iliac backbleeding is controlled with an occluding balloon cannula.

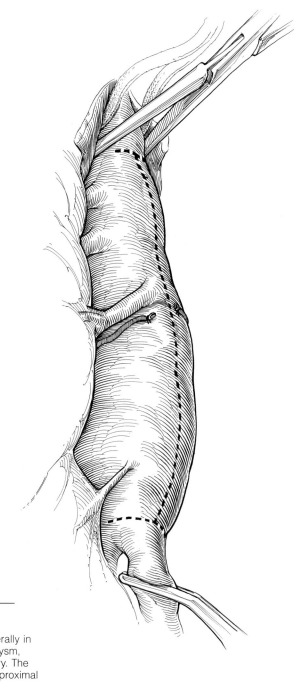

## Figure 126

The aortotomy is placed posterolaterally in this type 4 thoracoabdominal aneurysm, carefully avoiding the left renal artery. The incision is "T-ed" at the level of the proximal and distal anastomoses.

*Thoracoabdominal Aneurysm Repair*

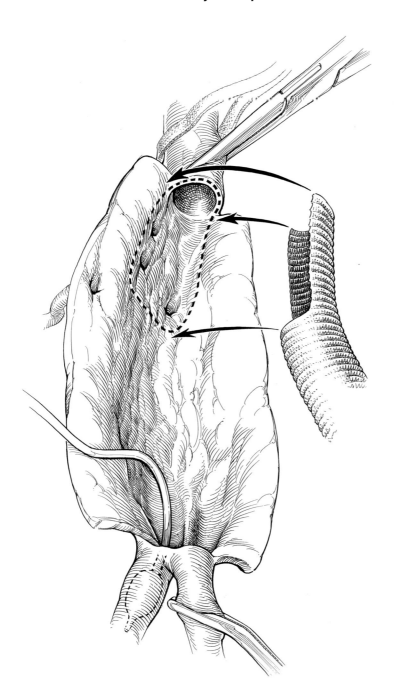

## Figure 127

The right iliac artery is controlled with balloon occlusion. The graft is beveled to allow inclusion of the celiac, superior mesenteric, and right renal orifices in the proximal anastomosis.

In a type 4 thoracoabdominal aneurysm, the celiac, mesenteric, and right renal orifices are included in a long, tapered, proximal anastomosis (Fig. 127). A woven polyester graft typically is used with 2-0 or 3-0 polypropylene sutures placed in a continuous fashion (Fig. 128). Thoracoabdominal aneurysms beginning in the chest require separate proximal and visceral anastomoses. In these cases, perfusion of the mesenteric and hepatic circulation during the construction of the proximal anastomosis may decrease coagulopathies, just as renal perfusion may limit the extent of postoperative azotemia. Many surgeons believe that reimplantation of intercoastal vessels is important in these aneurysms.

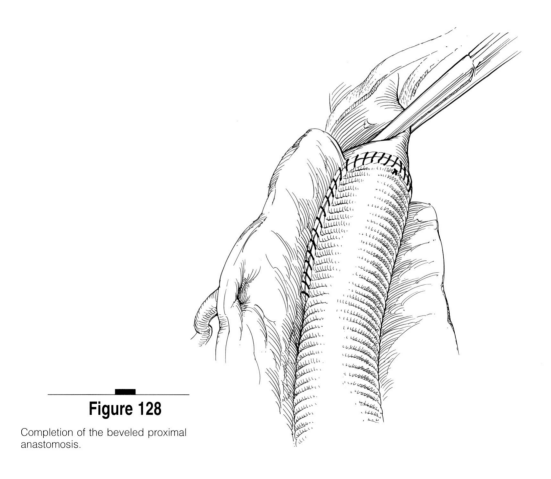

### Figure 128

Completion of the beveled proximal anastomosis.

## *Thoracoabdominal Aneurysm Repair*

The left renal artery is usually implanted separately onto the body of the graft (Fig. 129). This technique may cause the left renal artery to kink as the viscera are returned to their normal location. A separate graft limb may be used to bridge the defect between the left renal artery and the body of the aortic graft if this problem is encountered.

After the visceral anastomoses have been completed, the clamp is repositioned distally, gradually restoring prograde flow to the viscera, and the distal aortic anastomosis is performed with 3-0 polypropylene suture. Before placement of the last few sutures, the patient is placed in the head-down position, and the graft and native aorta are flushed to remove air and debris and to prevent embolization to the head.

When the anastomoses have been completed, the aneurysm sac is inspected for hemostasis. Particular attention is paid to lumbar vessels, which may begin backbleeding after distal perfusion has been restored. The aneurysm sac is then closed over the graft using a running stitch (Fig. 130). The diaphragm is then reapproximated, chest tubes are placed in the left chest for drainage, the chest and abdomen are closed, and the double-lumen endotracheal tube is changed to a standard tube for postoperative ventilatory support.

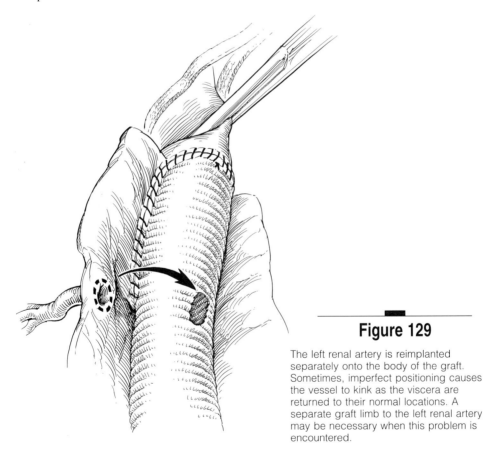

## Figure 129

The left renal artery is reimplanted separately onto the body of the graft. Sometimes, imperfect positioning causes the vessel to kink as the viscera are returned to their normal locations. A separate graft limb to the left renal artery may be necessary when this problem is encountered.

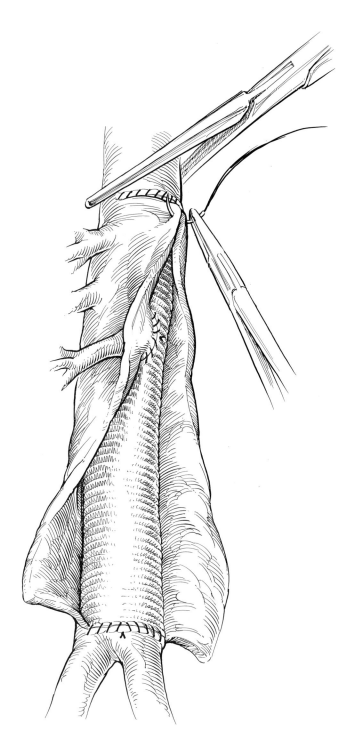

## Figure 130

The aneurysm sac is closed over the graft
on completion of the anastomoses.

# CHAPTER 19

# *Femoral Aneurysm Repair*

Femoral aneurysms have several forms. Native femoral artery aneurysms represent true aneurysms of the common femoral artery and are composed of all three layers of the normal arterial wall. *True femoral aneurysms* are frequently associated with aneurysms in other locations and are commonly seen in patients with diffuse arterial dilatation known as arteriomegally. *False femoral aneurysms* resulting from trauma represent organized hematomas bounded by a capsule of surrounding fibrous tissue. These aneurysms commonly are the result of iatrogenic injury, as occurs during interventional procedures such as peripheral thrombolytic therapy. An *anastomotic femoral aneurysm* is also relatively common and develops at the site of a graft to a femoral arterial anastomosis. They occur as the result of infection or mechanical disruption of the suture, graft, or arterial wall.

## OPERATIVE PROCEDURE

Repair of a true femoral artery aneurysm can be safely performed through a single, longitudinal groin incision unless the aneurysm extends proximally beneath the inguinal ligament. In that case, proximal control may be required through a separate retroperitoneal flank incision (Fig. 131). This approach provides controlled access to the external iliac artery (Fig. 132).

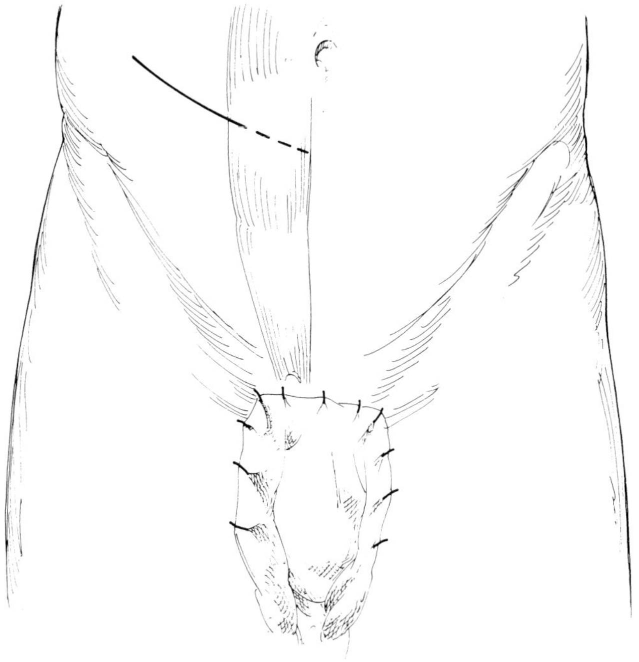

## Figure 131

The incision used for a retroperitoneal exposure of the right iliac system, performed as an initial step in the control of a high femoral aneurysm.

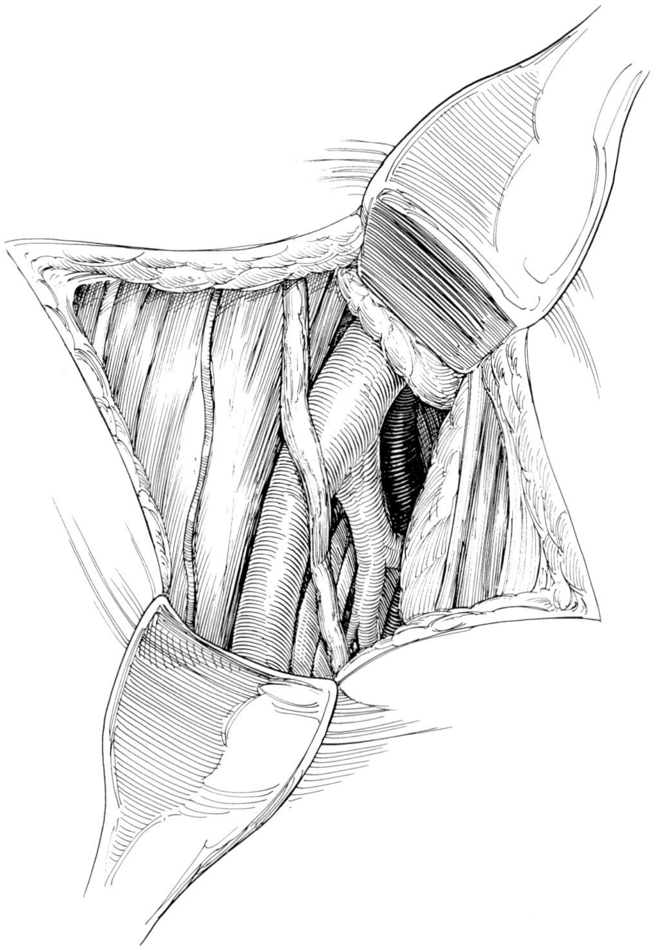

## Figure 132

The iliac vessels are exposed in the retroperitoneal space, and the external iliac artery is controlled just proximal to its exit beneath the inguinal ligament.

## Femoral Aneurysm Repair

It is important to gain control of the profunda femoris artery in addition to the distal external iliac artery and superficial femoral artery (Fig. 133). Profunda control is most easily achieved after control of the distal external iliac and superficial femoral arteries by retracting these vessels medially to allow dissection along the lateral surface of the aneurysm to reach the profunda femoris takeoff. Balloon occlusion catheters can be used when dense reaction makes dissection difficult. In these cases, the balloon catheter may be inserted proximally or distally to obtain control without complete dissection of the vessel.

Heparin is administered after the inflow and outflow vessels have been controlled. If the aneurysm ends sufficiently above the profunda origin, a simple prosthetic tube graft may be interposed, resecting the aneurysm in its entirety (Fig. 134). Alternatively, if the aneurysm ends are too close to the femoral bifurcation to perform a single distal anastomosis, a beveled, end-to-end anastomosis to the superficial femoral artery can be performed. The profunda femoral artery is reimplanted onto the side of the graft with 6-0 polypropylene suture (Fig. 135).

Other configurations are possible, including advancement of the common femoral bifurcation to a more distal level with a V-shaped anastomosis of the adjacent sides of the superficial femoral and profunda arteries together to form a conjoined orifice. When the femoral aneurysm is very large, the aneurysm may be left in situ, and the anastomoses can be sewn from within the aneurysmal sac in a manner analogous to that commonly employed when repairing an abdominal aortic aneurysm.

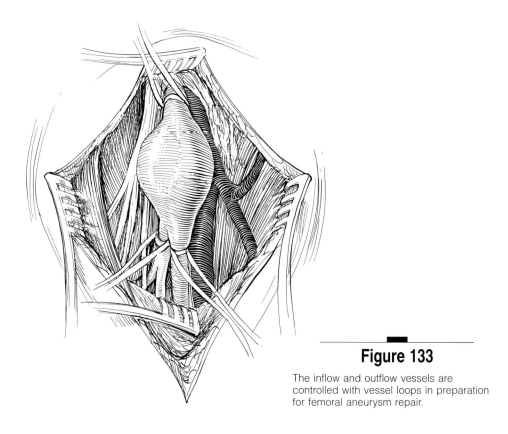

### Figure 133

The inflow and outflow vessels are controlled with vessel loops in preparation for femoral aneurysm repair.

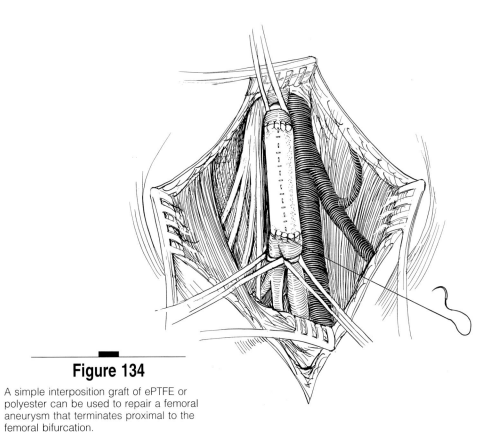

## Figure 134

A simple interposition graft of ePTFE or polyester can be used to repair a femoral aneurysm that terminates proximal to the femoral bifurcation.

## Figure 135

When the aneurysm extends to the femoral bifurcation, it is most efficient to bevel the graft and anastomose it directly to the superficial femoral artery in an end-to-end fashion. The profunda is then sewn to the side of the graft.

# CHAPTER 20

# Popliteal Aneurysm Repair Using a Posterior Approach

Popliteal aneurysms are found in saccular and fusiform configurations. *Saccular aneurysms* are prone to embolization, thrombosis, and compression of surrounding neural and venous structures. Although the more common *fusiform aneurysms* also embolize and frequently thrombose, their smaller size makes symptoms of neurologic and venous compression rare. Saccular aneurysms are usually confined to the popliteal fossa and are readily approached posteriorly with the patient in the prone position. Fusiform aneurysms generally begin in the superficial femoral artery and are probably more appropriately considered "femoropopliteal" aneurysms. Because this variety requires a medial approach—essentially a standard femoropopliteal bypass with exclusion by proximal and distal ligation of the involved vessels—it is not discussed further here.

## ▌ OPERATIVE PROCEDURE

The posterior approach to saccular popliteal aneurysm resection preferentially uses the saphenous vein for reconstruction if a prohibitive diameter mismatch does not exist. Preoperative vein mapping with duplex ultrasonography should be performed. If the lesser saphenous vein is inadequate, the greater saphenous vein is surprisingly easy to harvest with the patient in the prone position.

An S-shaped incision is made over the popliteal fossa, with the inferior portion of the incision directly overlying the lesser saphenous vein (Fig. 136). If adequate, the vein is excised from its superficial location at the mid-calf level to its deeper, subfascial location in the upper calf (Fig. 137A). The lesser saphenous vein enters the popliteal vein at various levels, and in many cases, the vein continues well above the popliteal skin crease to provide a much longer length of usable vein than otherwise expected. Venous branches are ligated with fine silk suture, and the vein is gently dilated and prepared as a reversed venous conduit (Fig. 137B).

The proximal, nonaneurysmal popliteal artery is located by palpation and controlled high in the popliteal fossa as it exits from the adductor canal. The artery is followed distally to its aneurysmal dilatation, being careful to avoid adherent and crossing veins. The aneurysm usually ends abruptly at the distal popliteal level, and the nonaneurysmal outflow is circumferentially controlled. There is no need to expose more than the most superficial portion of the aneurysm, which helps to avoid injury to adherent neurovascular structures.

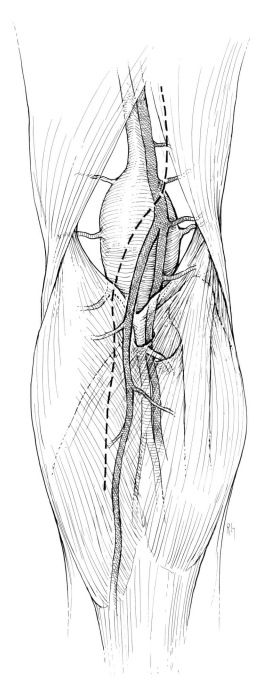

**Figure 136**

A lazy S–shaped incision is made, with the inferior margin placed over the lesser saphenous vein and the superior margin placed more medially. The lower portion of the vein lies superficially, and the upper portion runs beneath the investing fascia of the leg. The vein joins the popliteal vein at a variable level, sometimes well above the popliteal skin crease.

## Popliteal Aneurysm Repair Using a Posterior Approach

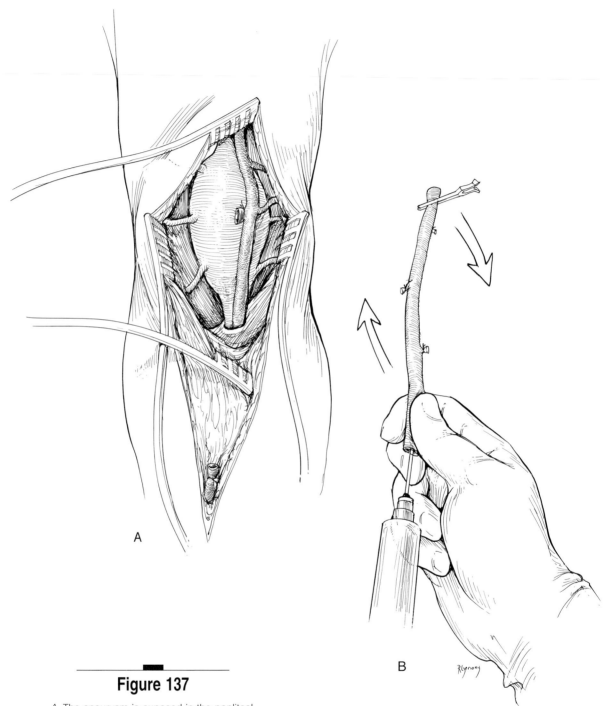

A

B

R.Gyrsony

### Figure 137

A, The aneurysm is exposed in the popliteal
fossa, taking care to avoid injury to the
adjacent popliteal veins and the tibial nerve.
B, The lesser saphenous vein is removed
and checked for leaks. The vein may be
used in a reversed or nonreversed manner.

After adequate heparinization, the popliteal artery is clamped above and below the aneurysm. The aneurysm is opened longitudinally, and geniculate branches are oversewn from within the aneurysm (Fig. 138A). The proximal anastomosis is performed in a beveled (Fig. 138B), end-to-end fashion using 6-0 polypropylene suture (Fig. 138C). Distally, a similar anastomosis is constructed. After release of the clamps, an adequate hemodynamic result is documented with a Doppler probe, duplex scanning, or intraoperative arteriography.

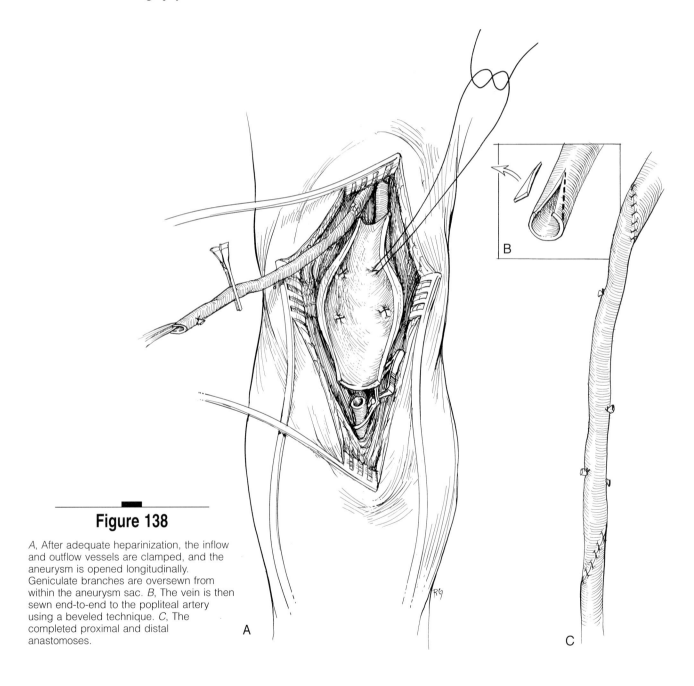

## Figure 138

*A,* After adequate heparinization, the inflow and outflow vessels are clamped, and the aneurysm is opened longitudinally. Geniculate branches are oversewn from within the aneurysm sac. *B,* The vein is then sewn end-to-end to the popliteal artery using a beveled technique. *C,* The completed proximal and distal anastomoses.

A

C

# RENAL AND VISCERAL ARTERIAL RECONSTRUCTION

# CHAPTER 21

# *Aortorenal Bypass*

Renal artery stenoses may result in renovascular hypertension and renal insuffi-ciency. Safer and more efficacious antihypertensive drugs have made control of the hypertensive complications of renal artery disease easier, but medical management of renovascular hypertension does not prevent progressive renal insufficiency from chronic hypoperfusion. Correction of significant renal artery narrowing (i.e., renal salvage sur-gery) can preserve functioning renal mass.

Diagnosis of a renovascular cause for hypertension or azotemia requires the clini-cian to be alert to the possibility and to order diagnostic tests to determine the anatomic location and functional significance of a stenotic lesion. We continue to rely on contrast arteriography to document the presence or absence of renal artery narrowing and use renal vein renin determinations when the functional significance of the lesion is in question. Duplex ultrasonography has gained increasing accuracy in the identification of renal artery stenoses. The determination relies on velocity elevations within a renal arterial stenosis and on the ratio of velocities within the renal artery relative to those in the aorta. Radionuclide imaging before and after provocative stimulation with the administration of angiotensin-converting enzyme inhibitors is gaining popularity as a screening test.

Because of the effects of a significant renal arterial lesion, there may not be enough functional renal mass to warrant salvage. The amount of functional cortex may be assessed by the use of computed tomography.

Renal arterial stenoses may be addressed with an endovascular or open surgical approach. Balloon angioplasty (i.e., percutaneous transluminal angioplasty) is effective for some nonostial lesions, particularly those resulting from fibromuscular dysplasia. Atherosclerotic lesions are commonly located at the origin of the renal artery and in continuity with dense plaque of the aortic wall. Balloon angioplasty has been ineffective in treating such ostial lesions. Stenting has been used to improve the results of percutane-ous transluminal angioplasty for ostial lesions, but long-term data showing efficacy are lacking.

Surgical renal artery reconstruction has involved endarterectomy or bypass. Endar-terectomy may be performed alone or at the time of aortic reconstruction for aneurysm or occlusive disease by carefully endarterectomizing the renal ostia through the open proximal aorta. In this technique of transaortic renal endarterectomy, mobilization of the proximal few centimeters of the renal arteries allows performance of an eversion endarterectomy. Because this is a somewhat blind approach, patency without defects must be confirmed after the procedure, usually with intraoperative duplex ultrasonography. Alternatively, a renal endarterectomy may be performed through a transverse incision extending from one renal artery onto the other. An open endarterectomy may then be performed with adequate visualization of the end point, but greater exposure is required. Renal endarterectomy is the procedure of choice when multiple renal arteries require reconstruction, especially in cases with coexistent accessory renal artery disease.

An acceptable algorithm for the treatment of renal artery disease can be summarized as follows:

1. Nonostial lesions are treated with balloon angioplasty, reserving placement of a stent for an unsatisfactory result, such as dissection or persistent stenosis.

2. Ostial lesions are treated with primary renal stenting when the patient is medically compromised.

3. In all other patients, ostial lesions are treated operatively, pending the availability of long-term follow-up data on stented patients.

4. Patients undergoing aortic procedures for coexistent aneurysmal or occlusive disease are treated with transaortic endarterectomy or bypass off the body of the aortic graft.

5. Patients with disease of unilateral renal disease and a relatively healthy aorta are treated with aortorenal bypass.

6. Patients with bilateral lesions or multiple renal artery lesions (i.e., main and accessory) should undergo endarterectomy if the aorta is clampable.

7. When the aorta is diseased and clamping would risk aortic injury or distal embolization, an extra-anatomic procedure is preferred. Acceptable sites of inflow include the splenic artery for left renal lesions, the hepatic artery for right renal lesions, or the iliac arteries when the celiac trunk or its branches are narrowed.

Renal artery bypass grafting offers some advantages over endarterectomy, especially when only one vessel is diseased. Problems associated with achieving a clean end point of the endarterectomy are avoided. Aortic clamping is limited to the infrarenal aortic segment or, in the case of hepatorenal and splenorenal extra-anatomic procedures, is not required at all.

## OPERATIVE PROCEDURE

**Primary Aortorenal Bypass.** Standard aortorenal bypass, used to treat patients with minimal disease of the infrarenal aortic segment, is performed through a midline transperitoneal or left retroperitoneal approach. In either case, the left renal artery is most easily exposed with medial displacement of the left colon and spleen (Fig. 139), and the right renal artery is most easily approached with right medial visceral rotation (Fig. 140). After careful mobilization and retraction of the renal vein, the renal artery is cleared of surrounding tissue.

*Aortorenal Bypass*

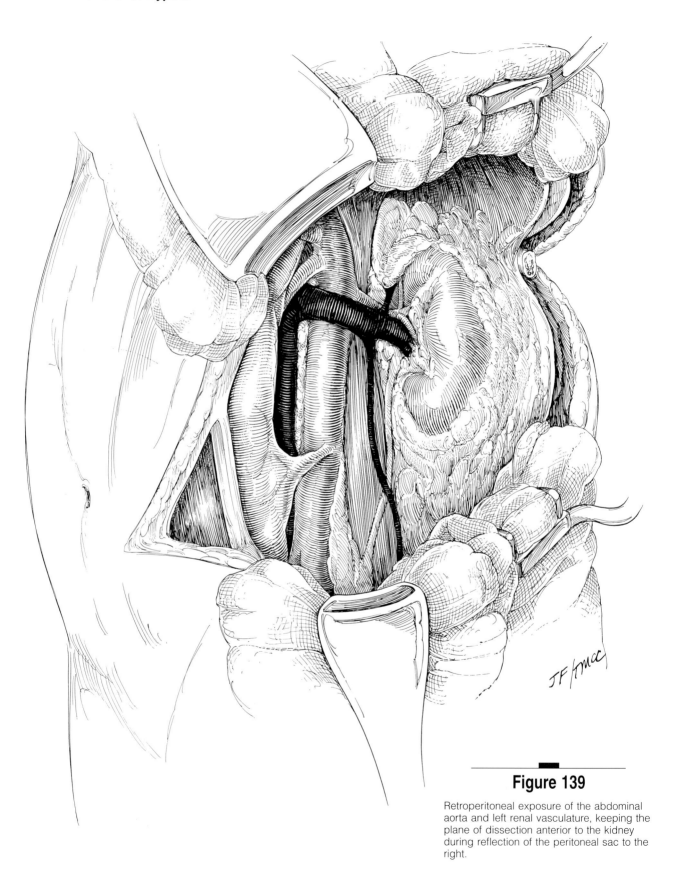

**Figure 139**

Retroperitoneal exposure of the abdominal
aorta and left renal vasculature, keeping the
plane of dissection anterior to the kidney
during reflection of the peritoneal sac to the
right.

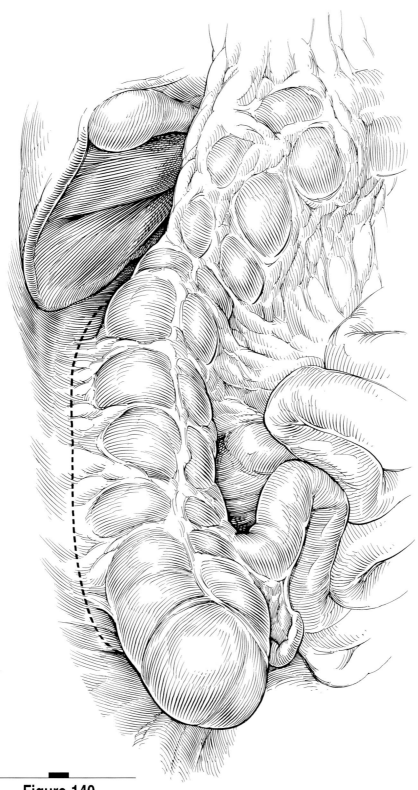

**Figure 140**

Reflection of the right colon to expose the
right renal hilum.

## *Aortorenal Bypass*

The aorta is palpated for disease, and if disease is unexpectedly extensive, the use of aortic inflow is abandoned and an alternative (usually extra-anatomic) procedure is chosen. Otherwise, the patient is administered heparin, and proximal and distal aortic clamps are applied (Fig. 141). An oblique orientation of the distal clamp obviates the need to control individual lumbar vessels. The use of a side-biting clamp is not advised. An ellipse should be removed from the aortic wall with the scissors or with multiple applications of an aortic punch.

Prosthetic or autogenous conduits have been used with long-term success. We favor the use of a saphenous vein graft, except in the pediatric population, in whom it is prone to aneurysmal degeneration. Hypogastric arterial grafts provide an acceptable alternative in children, although reimplantation of the renal artery onto the aorta is becoming the preferred treatment in very young patients.

The proximal and distal anastomoses are performed with 5-0 or 6-0 polypropylene suture (Fig. 142), carefully adjusting for length between anastomoses to avoid angulation and kinking. The patency of the reconstruction is assessed with duplex ultrasonography after removing the clamps. A fall or stabilization in the serum creatinine level can be anticipated, but resolution of hypertension is neither uniform nor dramatic. Although most patients require fewer antihypertensive agents after the procedure, complete resolution of hypertension is rare in those for whom the indication was renal salvage; complete resolution is observed mostly in younger patients with recent-onset hypertension. Duplex ultrasonography is used for postoperative surveillance of the graft.

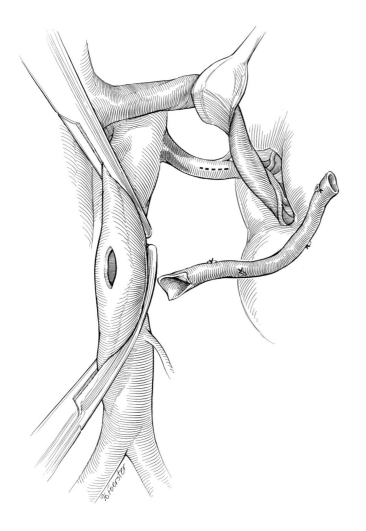

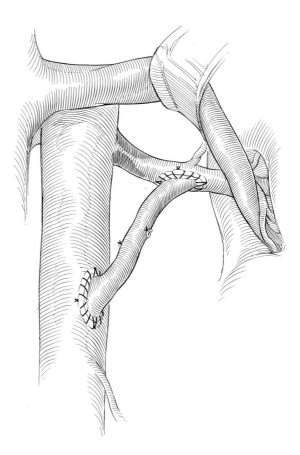

## Figure 141

When minimally diseased, the aorta is used as the site of inflow. Saphenous vein from the upper thigh or a prosthetic graft may be used. Proximal and distal aortic clamps are applied as shown. The proximal anastomosis is completed with polypropylene suture. The renal vein is retracted to expose a suitable length of renal artery, and the distal anastomosis is constructed with 6-0 polypropylene suture.

## Figure 142

The completed bypass should lie free in the retroperitoneal space without kinking or twisting of the graft.

## Aortorenal Bypass

**Aortorenal Bypass in Conjunction With Aortic Procedures.** A significant renal artery lesion coexisting with an abdominal aortic aneurysm (Fig. 143) or severe aortoiliac occlusive disease tempts the surgeon to correct the renal problem in conjunction with the aortic procedure. However, the morbidity of the aortic procedure is definitely increased by addition of a renal reconstruction. Simultaneous procedures should be considered only in reasonable-risk patients with significant renovascular hypertension or renal insufficiency.

The proximal left renal artery is approached after mobilization and retraction of the left renal vein through extension of the same exposure used for the aorta. Alternatively, more distal exposure of the artery may be easier after medial displacement of the left colon and spleen. Exposure of the distal right renal artery is easier after medial rotation of the right colon and duodenum, because the vena cava obscures all but the proximal portion of the vessel when approached through the same exposure used for the aorta.

A side limb (6- to 8-mm polyester or ePTFE) is sewn to the body of the aortic graft with 5-0 or 6-0 polypropylene suture. This can be done early, usually on the back table during the anesthesia induction when the renal artery bypass is part of the preoperative plan. The aortic reconstruction is then carried out in the usual fashion, with a clamp on the renal side limb. After completion of the aortic anastomoses, the renal anastomosis is performed using 6-0 polypropylene suture for joining this side limb to a convenient segment of renal artery free of disease (Fig. 144).

An adequate technical result is confirmed with duplex ultrasonography. The aneurysm sac is closed over the graft, fashioning a short slit to allow the renal graft to remain in proper position. Postoperatively, patency of the renal graft is monitored using color duplex ultrasonography.

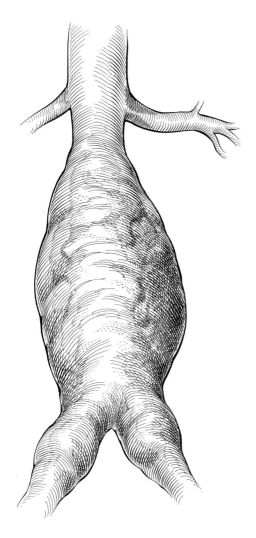

## Figure 143

Concomitant aneurysm resection (or aortobifemoral bypass for occlusive disease) and renal artery bypass may be appropriate when the renal lesion is causing symptoms of hypertension or renal insufficiency.

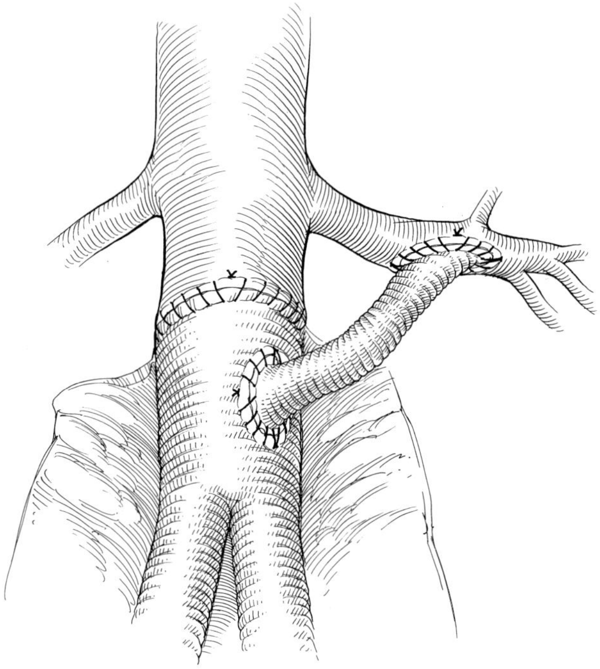

## Figure 144

After completion of the aortic anastomoses, a side limb is anastomosed to the renal artery at a point beyond the diseased area.

# CHAPTER 22

# Extra-anatomic Renal Revascularization

The frequent association of extensive abdominal aortic atherosclerotic disease with renal artery stenosis has led to the use of extra-anatomic renal revascularization. On the left side, a splenorenal bypass may be constructed by anastomosing the end of the splenic artery to the left renal artery. On the right side, a hepatorenal bypass is appropriate, employing an autogenous or prosthetic graft to bypass from the hepatic artery to the right renal artery. In each case, the application of an aortic clamp is avoided, greatly reducing the risks of aortic injury or distal embolization. The hemodynamic consequences of aortic clamping also are avoided—an important advantage in the medically compromised patient. Applicability of the procedure, however, is limited to those without occlusive lesions in the celiac artery or its splenic and hepatic branches leading to the bypass site.

## OPERATIVE PROCEDURE

**Splenorenal Bypass.** A splenorenal bypass is performed through a left subcostal or a midline abdominal incision. The left renal artery is approached after a medial visceral rotation, although an approach through the lesser sac is also appropriate.

The spleen and left colon are mobilized from their retroperitoneal attachments by carefully dividing the splenocolic bands to prevent injury to the splenic capsule (Fig. 145). The spleen and left colon are then elevated anteromedially, leaving the left kidney undisturbed by keeping the plane of dissection anterior to Gerota's fascia. The left renal vein is usually the first structure to be identified within the fatty retroperitoneal tissues between the aorta and the left renal hilum. The vein is gently mobilized, being careful to avoid injury to the adrenal or gonadal veins. Division of the adrenal branch and caudal retraction of the left renal vein expose the left renal artery.

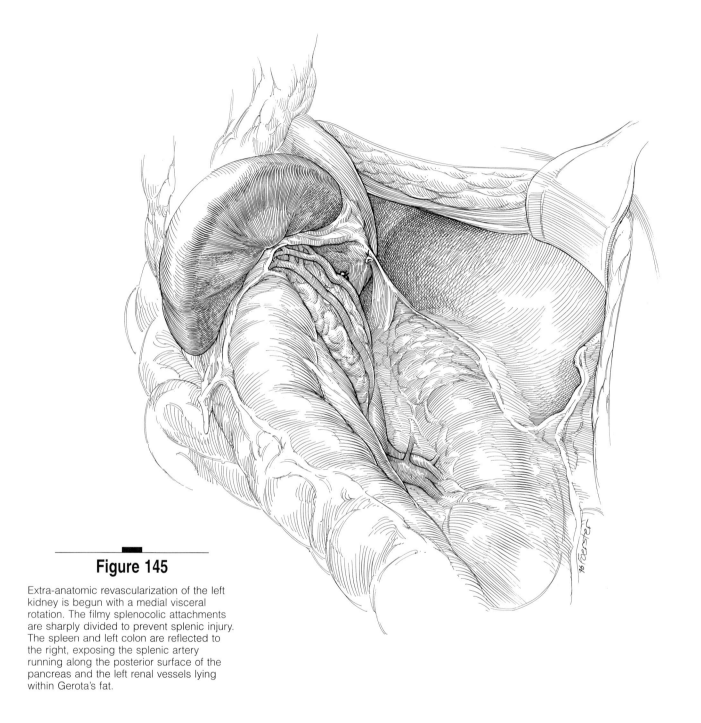

## Figure 145

Extra-anatomic revascularization of the left kidney is begun with a medial visceral rotation. The filmy splenocolic attachments are sharply divided to prevent splenic injury. The spleen and left colon are reflected to the right, exposing the splenic artery running along the posterior surface of the pancreas and the left renal vessels lying within Gerota's fat.

## Extra-anatomic Renal Revascularization

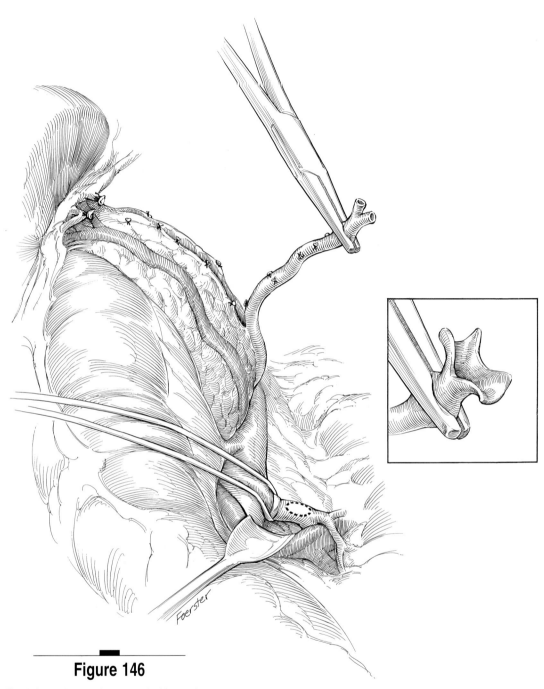

Foerster

### Figure 146

The left renal artery is exposed with gentle
inferior retraction of the renal vein. The
splenic artery is mobilized as far as
necessary to provide an adequate length to
reach the left renal artery. The artery can be
divided just beyond its major bifurcation to
allow the creation of a larger ostium for
anastomosis *(inset)*.

Palpation at the splenic hilum allows the surgeon to locate the splenic artery. The artery is dissected circumferentially and followed proximally along the posterior aspect of the pancreas to obtain adequate length. Small arterial branches between the splenic artery and the substance of the pancreas must be carefully ligated and divided (Fig. 146). The spleen need not be removed unless it is injured, because the short gastric arteries provide adequate blood flow to maintain viability. The splenic artery may be heavily calcified and tortuous, and occasionally, a localized eversion endarterectomy of the distal vessel may be necessary to obtain a pliable conduit suitable for clamping and anastomosis.

The patient is administered heparin, and the splenic artery is transected at its bifurcation near the splenic hilum. If the artery is divided just beyond a point of major branching, the branches can be incised to provide a larger orifice for anastomosis (see Fig. 146, *inset*). The renal artery is occluded, and an end-to-end or end-to-side anastomosis is constructed between the splenic artery and the left renal artery (Fig. 147). At the conclusion of this anastomosis, patency is ascertained with the use of an intraoperative Doppler or duplex ultrasonography. The spleen and viscera are then returned to their normal positions, and the subcostal incision is closed.

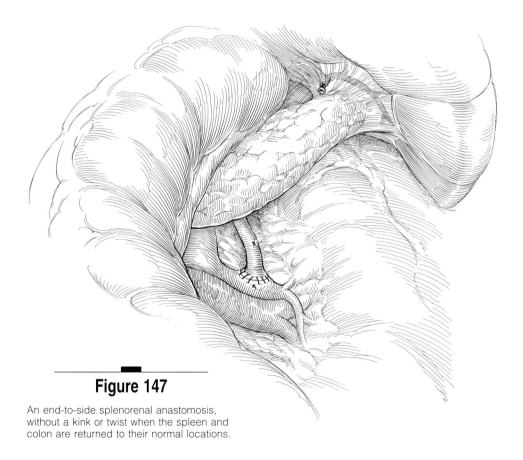

## Figure 147

An end-to-side splenorenal anastomosis,
without a kink or twist when the spleen and
colon are returned to their normal locations.

## *Extra-anatomic Renal Revascularization*

**Hepatorenal Bypass.** Like the splenorenal bypass, a hepatorenal bypass allows performance of a renal arterial reconstruction without clamping a heavily diseased abdominal aorta. A right subcostal or midline abdominal incision is used. When bilateral renal revascularization is necessary, a hepatorenal bypass may be performed in conjunction with a splenorenal bypass through a long chevron incision.

After incision of the lateral attachments of the right colon and hepatic flexure, exposure commences with reflection of the right colon and duodenum to the left and performance of a Kocher maneuver (Fig. 148). The right renal vein is the first structure to be visualized, and gentle caudal retraction of the vein exposes the right renal artery.

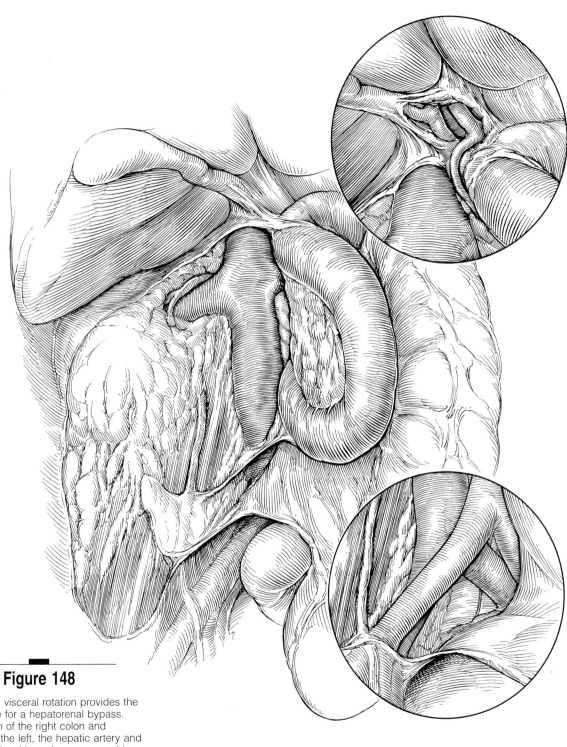

**Figure 148**

A right medial visceral rotation provides the
best exposure for a hepatorenal bypass.
After reflection of the right colon and
duodenum to the left, the hepatic artery and
its gastroduodenal branch are exposed in
the lesser omentum *(upper inset)*. When
significant celiac disease precludes the use
of hepatic inflow, the right iliac system is
easily exposed using this approach *(lower
inset)*.

## *Extra-anatomic Renal Revascularization*

The hepatic artery is palpated in the lesser omentum, just medial to the common bile duct. A hepatic artery "thrill" often is palpable, even in the absence of stenosis, because of its high resting flow. The junction of the common and proper hepatic arteries is dissected free of surrounding tissue, along with a proximal portion of the gastroduodenal artery (Fig. 149). Alternatively, the iliac system can provide an acceptable source of inflow if the celiac trunk is diseased. Mobilization of the cecum provides easy access to the vessel, running the graft parallel to the ureter to reach the renal hilum.

A suitable length of conduit is harvested. Approximately 15 cm of greater saphenous vein usually is required, but an externally supported ePTFE graft may also be appropriate (Fig. 150). The patient is administered heparin, and the common hepatic, proper hepatic, and gastroduodenal vessels are occluded with vessel loops. A longitudinal arteriotomy is made, beginning on the common hepatic artery and extending to the proper hepatic

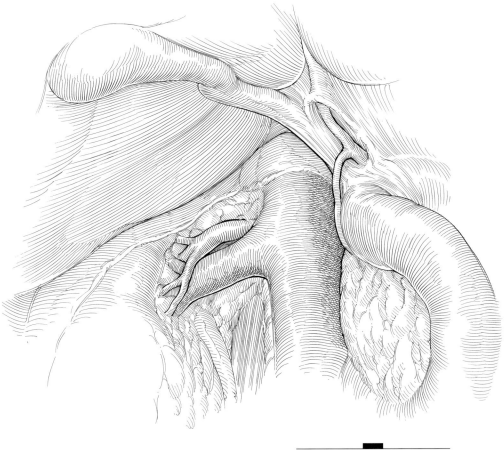

## Figure 149

The exposed right renal artery and hepatic artery with its gastroduodenal branch.

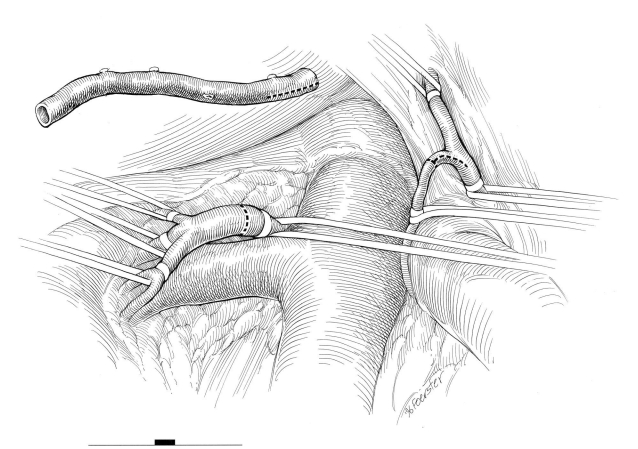

## Figure 150

After harvest of an adequate length of
greater saphenous vein from the upper
thigh, the patient is heparinized, and the
vessels are occluded. The hepatic
arteriotomy is made along the main portion
of the vessel; alternatively, the arteriotomy is
carried onto the gastroduodenal artery.

## Extra-anatomic Renal Revascularization

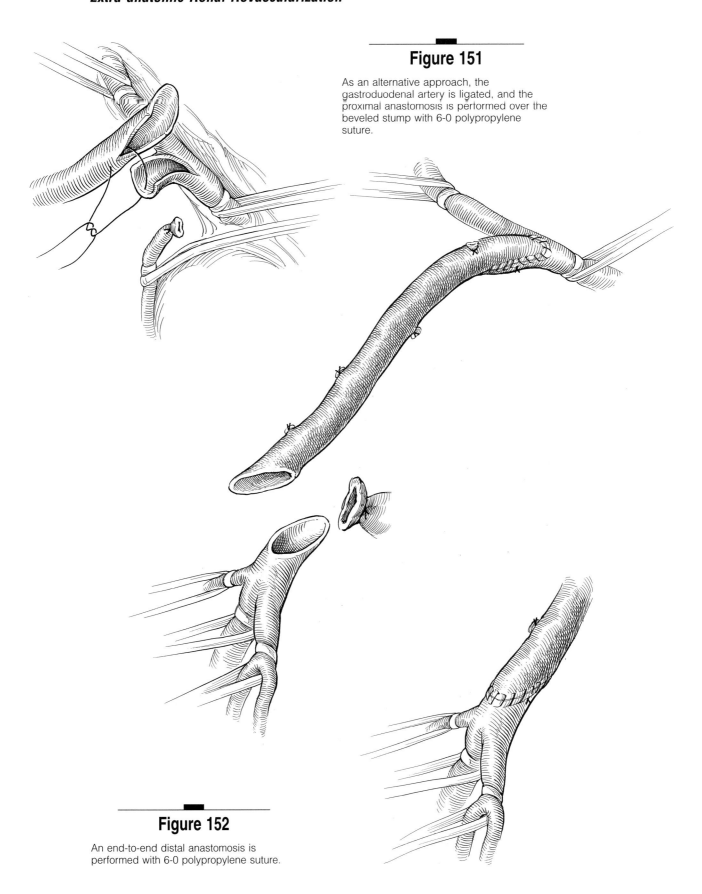

### Figure 151

As an alternative approach, the gastroduodenal artery is ligated, and the proximal anastomosis is performed over the beveled stump with 6-0 polypropylene suture.

### Figure 152

An end-to-end distal anastomosis is performed with 6-0 polypropylene suture.

artery. Alternatively, the gastroduodenal artery can be ligated and divided, leaving a short stump suitable for anastomosis (Fig. 151). The proximal anastomosis is constructed with 6-0 polypropylene suture. The distal anastomosis is then performed in an end-to-end or end-to-side fashion using 6-0 polypropylene suture (Fig. 152).

After the anastomoses have been completed (Fig. 153), patency is ascertained with intraoperative Doppler or duplex ultrasonography. On returning the viscera to their normal positions, the surgeon must be certain that the graft does not kink. The subcostal wound is closed in layers.

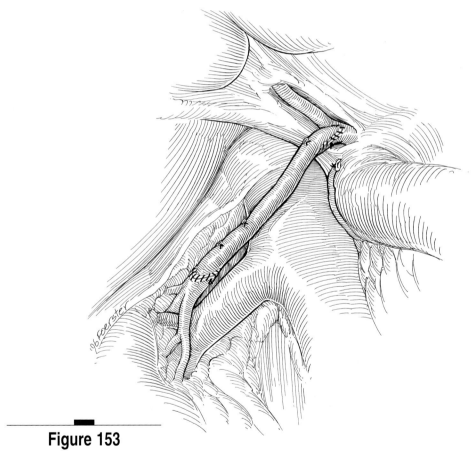

## Figure 153

The completed hepatorenal bypass, lying without a kink or twist as the viscera are returned to their normal locations.

# CHAPTER 23

# Mesenteric Arterial Bypass

Chronic mesenteric occlusive disease commonly becomes symptomatic when the celiac axis and the superior mesenteric artery (SMA) inflow are significantly narrowed or occluded. Disease of only one of the two vessels is rarely associated with postprandial pain severe enough to create "food fear." Patients typically present in an emaciated state, and the absence of significant weight loss should make the diagnosis suspect. Although color duplex ultrasonography can confirm the diagnosis, it requires an experienced technician. Contrast arteriography is therefore the diagnostic procedure of choice and is performed with lateral views to demonstrate the origins of the celiac axis and SMA.

Multivessel occlusive disease associated with the clinical picture of chronic mesenteric ischemia mandates revascularization of the celiac axis and the SMA. A short, antegrade reconstruction can provide a better hemodynamic result than a long, retrograde bypass. It is best to position the proximal anastomosis of the graft on the supraceliac aorta, rather than placing the anastomosis infrarenally and running the graft in a retrograde direction. The advantage of an antegrade reconstruction does not mean that a well-constructed retrograde procedure is never appropriate. Under certain circumstances, a retrograde bypass may be the procedure of choice, as for most cases of acute mesenteric thromboses.

## OPERATIVE PROCEDURE

**Anterior Approach to Mesenteric Bypass.** Antegrade bypass to the celiac and superior mesenteric arterial beds is begun with exposure of the supraceliac, infradiaphragmatic aorta. The approach is essentially an extended version of that used to gain emergency control of that segment, as described in *Atlas of Vascular Surgery: Basic Techniques and Exposures.* Through a midline transperitoneal approach, the triangular ligament is divided, and the left lobe of the liver is reflected to the right. A rent is made in the lesser omentum while palpating the nasogastric tube to locate the esophagus and avoid injury. The crura of the diaphragm are divided, and the supraceliac aorta is exposed (Fig. 154).

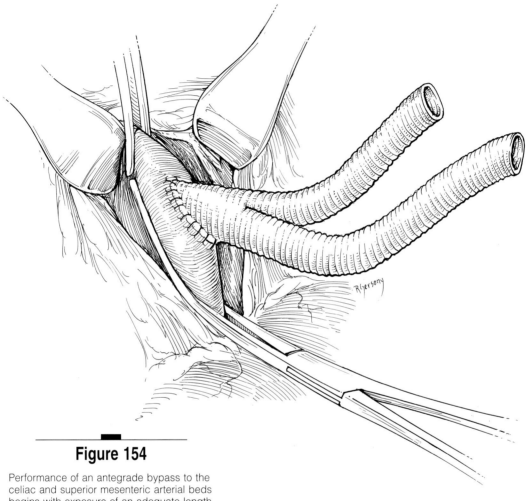

## Figure 154

Performance of an antegrade bypass to the celiac and superior mesenteric arterial beds begins with exposure of an adequate length of supraceliac aorta. A midline abdominal, transperitoneal approach is employed. The triangular ligament is incised, and the left lobe of the liver is reflected to the right. The crura are divided, and the aorta is cleared from the celiac axis to a proximal level within the lower mediastinum.

## Mesenteric Arterial Bypass

In contrast to the relatively short length of supraceliac aorta exposure necessary for application of a clamp, a long length must be cleared for the performance of an anastomosis. Continued dissection along the anterior surface of the aorta into the mediastinum provides a relatively straightforward means of obtaining an adequate length. The patient's emaciated state makes this exposure surprisingly easy.

Although the proximal celiac artery may be exposed at the distal aspect of the field in cases of stenoses, in cases of occlusion, access to the celiac arterial bed is most easily accomplished by exposing the hepatic artery in the lesser omentum (Fig. 155). Although the artery is usually pulseless in this group of patients, the lack of fatty tissue renders its location readily apparent.

The SMA is exposed at the root of the mesentery. Leaving the small bowel down and reflecting the transverse colon cranially provides anterior access to the midportion of the vessel. Alternatively, the small bowel can be reflected to the right, and the ligament of Treitz is incised to provide access to the more proximal portion of the SMA as it runs behind the pancreas (Fig. 156). Although it is more technically demanding, we prefer the latter approach, because of the larger diameter at the SMA outflow site.

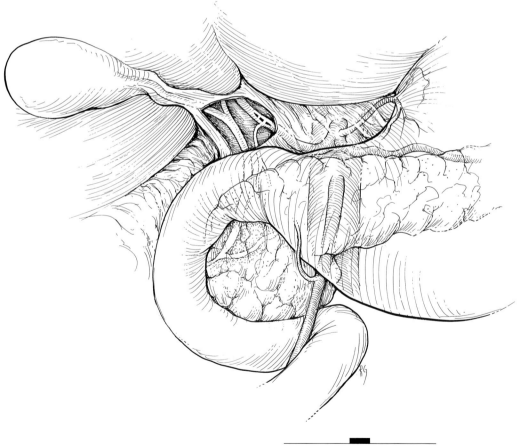

## Figure 155

The common hepatic artery is exposed within the lesser omentum.

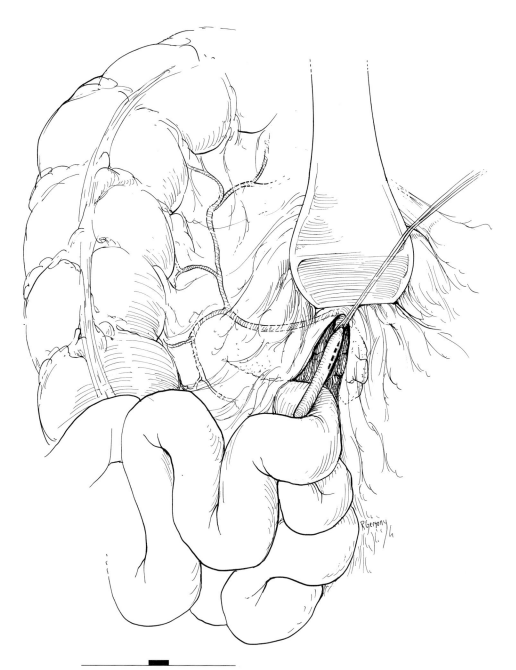

**Figure 156**

The ligament of Treitz is incised and the duodenum is reflected to the right. The superior mesenteric artery is exposed as it runs along the posterior surface of the pancreas to cross the duodenum.

## Mesenteric Arterial Bypass

A small-diameter bifurcated polyester or ePTFE graft is chosen; it is usually 12 × 6 mm or 14 × 7 mm. The body of the graft is cut very short and beveled appropriately. No tunnel is necessary for the short right (hepatic artery) graft limb, because it lies on the surface of the lesser omentum. The tunnel to the SMA runs posterior to the pancreas and is created with careful digital dissection in a plane anterior to the aorta and just to the left of the celiac and superior mesenteric vessels.

After systemic heparinization, the supraceliac aorta is clamped proximally and distally. The proximal graft anastomosis is constructed with 3-0 or 4-0 polypropylene suture (Fig. 157). The distal anastomoses are completed with 5-0 or 6-0 suture. Care must be exercised in planning the SMA anastomosis to avoid twisting the graft as the small bowel is returned to its normal location.

Duplex ultrasonography is used to ensure technical success after completion of the anastomoses. Heparin is reversed with protamine sulfate, if needed, and the wound is closed.

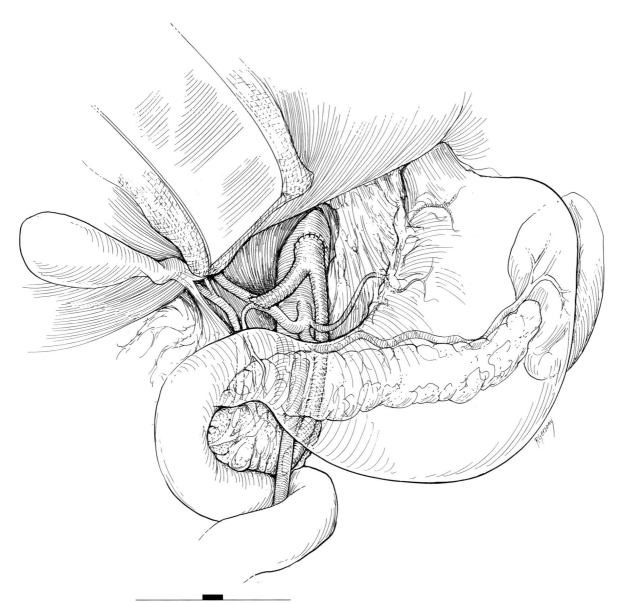

## Figure 157

A bifurcated polyester prosthesis is
employed, usually 12 × 6 mm or 14 × 7
mm. The proximal anastomosis is
constructed to the supraceliac aorta using
3-0 or 4-0 polypropylene suture. The short
hepatic graft limb is anastomosed to the
side of the common hepatic artery using 5-0
or 6-0 suture. The superior mesenteric
artery (SMA) graft limb is tunneled behind
the pancreas, running just lateral to the
celiac trunk. The SMA anastomosis is
performed in an end-to-side manner,
avoiding twisting of the graft limb as the
viscera are returned to their normal
locations.

## Mesenteric Arterial Bypass

**Mesenteric Bypass Using a Medial Visceral Rotation.** An alternative approach to proximal celiac and superior mesenteric disease involves medial visceral rotation, reflecting the spleen and tail of the pancreas to the right and leaving the left kidney in place (Fig. 158). The crus of the diaphragm is incised, and the proximal celiac axis and SMA are exposed (Fig. 159). If the celiac plaque is adequately localized, a limited endarterectomy may be accomplished (Fig. 160). The aortotomy can then be used as the inflow site for a single graft to the SMA (Fig. 161). The proximal anastomosis of the bypass graft effectively functions as a patch angioplasty of the proximal celiac axis. An 8-mm or 10-mm polyester graft is usually appropriate, using 4-0 or 5-0 polypropylene suture for the proximal anastomosis and 6-0 suture distally.

This approach is not possible when the aortic disease is severe at the celiac level. In that case, the inflow originates from a separate aortotomy placed more proximally, using a bifurcated graft to the celiac trunk and SMA (Fig. 162) or a single graft with an end-to-side celiac to graft anastomosis and an end-to-end SMA anastomosis (Fig. 163).

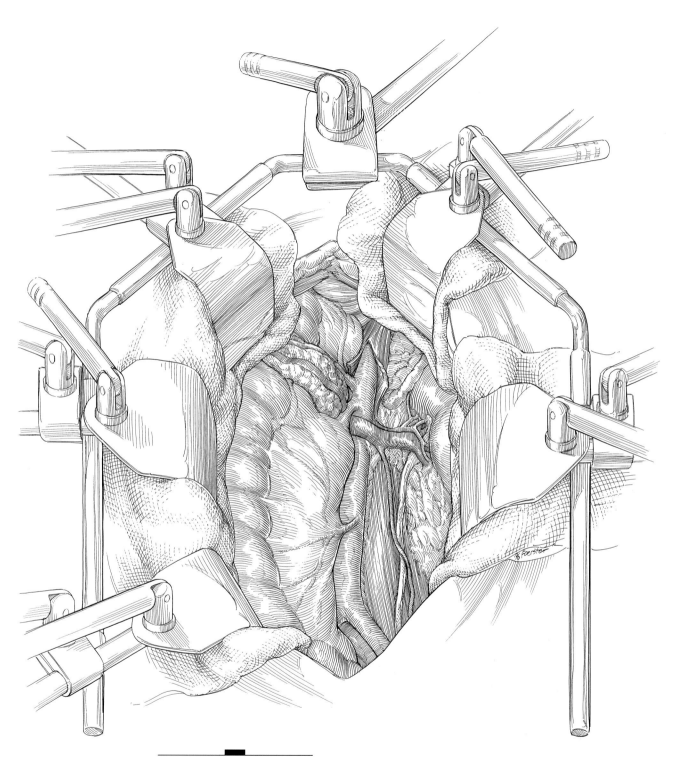

**Figure 158**

Exposure of the abdominal aorta using a
medial visceral rotation. The crura of the
diaphragm are incised to obtain additional
supraceliac aortic length.

## Mesenteric Arterial Bypass

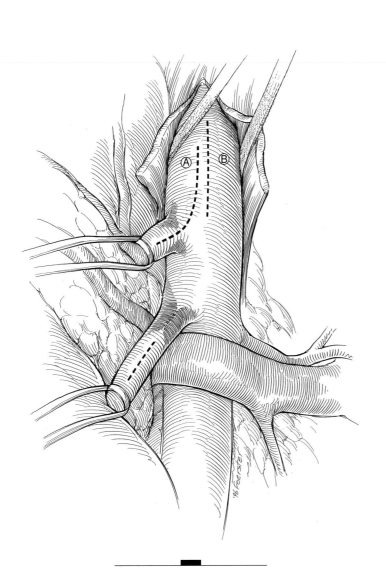

**Figure 159**

A medial visceral rotation affords direct access to the celiac and superior mesenteric artery origins. When the celiac disease is localized, the aortotomy may be carried distally onto the celiac trunk itself (*A*), with the proximal graft anastomosis functioning as a patch angioplasty of the celiac lesion. Alternatively, the aortotomy may be kept on the supraceliac aorta (*B*), and two separate distal anastomoses are performed.

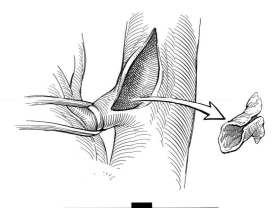

**Figure 160**

When the plaque is localized, an endarterectomy is feasible.

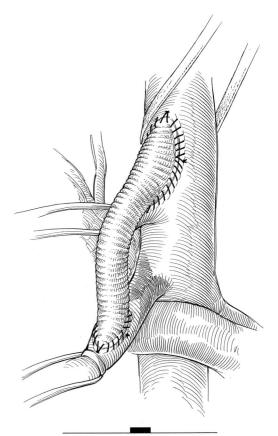

**Figure 161**

After endarterectomy of the celiac orifice, the graft is sewn in place. Proximally, the anastomosis is performed with 5-0 polypropylene suture; distally, 6-0 suture is employed.

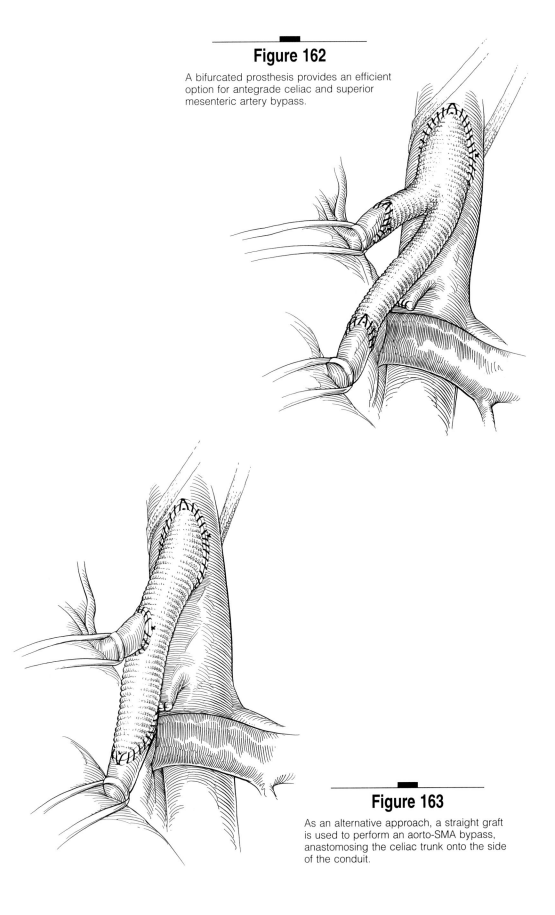

### Figure 162

A bifurcated prosthesis provides an efficient option for antegrade celiac and superior mesenteric artery bypass.

### Figure 163

As an alternative approach, a straight graft is used to perform an aorto-SMA bypass, anastomosing the celiac trunk onto the side of the conduit.

## Mesenteric Arterial Bypass

**Superior Mesenteric Artery Reimplantation.** When bowel resection may be necessary, it is advisable to refrain from the use of a prosthetic graft in patients with acute mesenteric ischemia. A single-vessel (i.e., SMA) reconstruction is an acceptable option in this setting.

After medial visceral rotation, the SMA is exposed at its junction with the aorta, just cephalad to the left renal vein (Fig. 164). The SMA is dissected free of surrounding tissue for a distance of several centimeters, and the first few small duodenal branches are ligated and divided. The left renal vein is mobilized and retracted in a cephalad direction, and the SMA is divided, followed by oversewing the proximal stump (Fig. 165). The aorta is clamped, and an aortotomy is made with a No. 11 knife (Fig. 166). The aortotomy may be extended into a circular defect using a punch (Fig. 167), and an anastomosis of an end of the SMA to the side of the aorta is fashioned with 5-0 or 6-0 polypropylene suture (Fig. 168). The renal vein is then returned to its normal location (Fig. 169), and patency of reconstruction confirmed by the presence of a full pulse without a thrill.

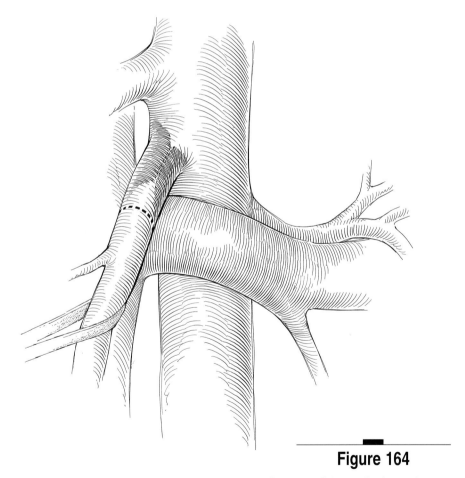

### Figure 164

Exposure of the proximal superior mesenteric artery (SMA) and pararenal aorta in preparation for reimplantation of the SMA.

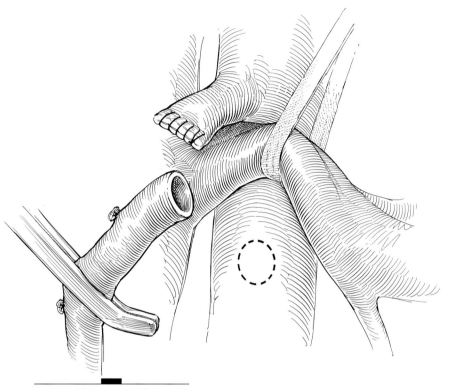

**Figure 165**

The superior mesenteric artery is divided,
and the proximal stump is oversewn.

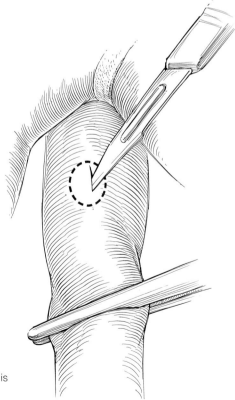

**Figure 166**

The aorta is clamped, and an anterior slit is
made with a No. 11 knife.

## Mesenteric Arterial Bypass

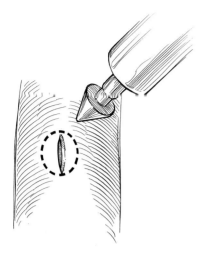

### Figure 167

The slit is extended into a circular ostium with the aid of an aortic punch.

### Figure 168

An end-to-side anastomosis is constructed with 5-0 or 6-0 polypropylene suture.

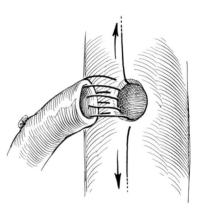

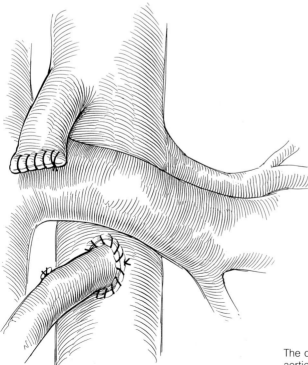

### Figure 169

The completed superior mesenteric artery to aortic anastomosis.

**Retrograde Superior Mesenteric Artery Revascularization.** A retrograde approach to superior mesenteric arterial reconstruction involves the use of the infrarenal aorta for inflow. In addition to the theoretical disadvantage of retrograde blood flow, kinking of the graft is a major drawback. After the viscera are returned to their normal locations, a saphenous vein or unsupported prosthetic conduit may kink, resulting in immediate failure of the reconstruction (Fig. 170).

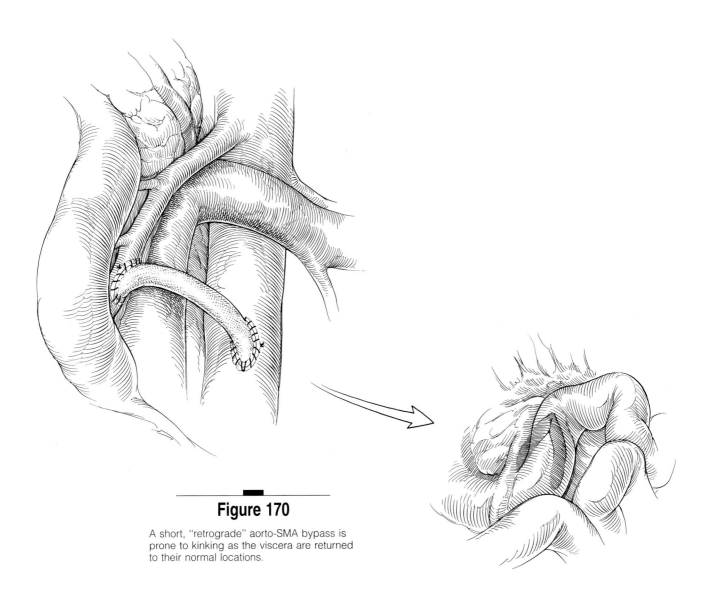

**Figure 170**

A short, "retrograde" aorto-SMA bypass is prone to kinking as the viscera are returned to their normal locations.

## *Mesenteric Arterial Bypass*

An alternative is an externally supported ePTFE graft. A greater length of 6-mm prosthesis is employed (Fig. 171), with the surgeon positioning the proximal and distal anastomoses on the distal infrarenal aorta and SMA, respectively. The longer graft makes a gentle arc as the viscera are returned to their normal locations, and kinking of the prosthesis is prevented. This longer configuration is associated with patency rates similar to those for antegrade bypass.

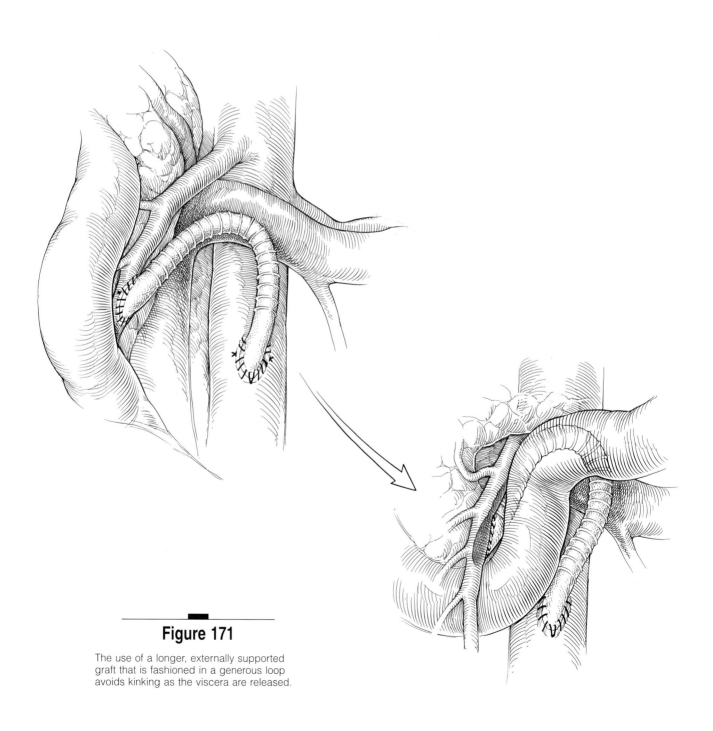

### Figure 171

The use of a longer, externally supported graft that is fashioned in a generous loop avoids kinking as the viscera are released.

**Trap Door Aortic Endarterectomy for Visceral and Renal Artery Occlusive Disease.** Diffuse atheromatous disease of the proximal abdominal aorta may compromise the visceral and renal vessels (Fig. 172). As an alternative to separate reconstruction of each involved vessel, Dr. G. Melville Williams proposed a trap door approach, with the use of visceral and renal endarterectomy. The procedure requires an aorta that is clampable at the supraceliac and infrarenal levels, and the disease in the mesenteric or renal arteries must not extend beyond the first 1 to 2 cm. Localized ostial involvement is common when the primary process is that of aortic atherosclerosis.

The aorta is exposed retroperitoneally or through a transperitoneal approach with medial visceral rotation. When the retroperitoneal approach is used, the surgeon may still need to enter the peritoneal cavity after the reconstruction to ascertain viability of the intestine.

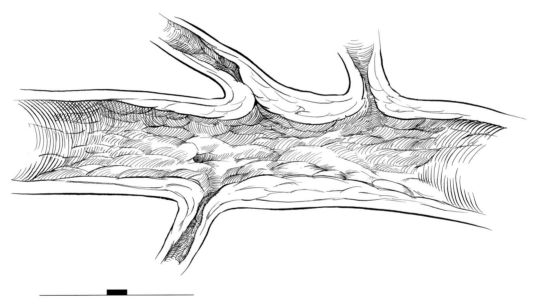

## Figure 172

Atherosclerotic disease causing ostial stenoses of multiple visceral vessels is a condition amenable to a trap door aortic endarterectomy. The aorta must be clampable above and below this level, and the branch vessel disease must be limited to the first 1 or 2 cm of each vessel.

## Mesenteric Arterial Bypass

After an adequate length of aorta has been exposed, the left renal, superior mesenteric, and celiac takeoffs are dissected free of surrounding tissue. After heparin is administered, the aorta is clamped proximally and distally, and a trap door arteriotomy is made (Fig. 173). An endarterectomy plane is established, reflecting the aortic outer media and adventitia to the right (Fig. 174). A blind eversion endarterectomy is performed, involving the celiac trunk, SMA, and right renal artery. An endarterectomy of the left renal artery is performed (Fig. 175), and the aortotomy is closed with a running 4-0 or 5-0 polypropylene suture. A distal intimal flap is rarely a problem, and tacking sutures are only occasionally employed.

Patency of the involved vessels is established intraoperatively with Doppler or duplex ultrasonography. After inspection of the bowel, the abdominal wound is closed in a standard fashion.

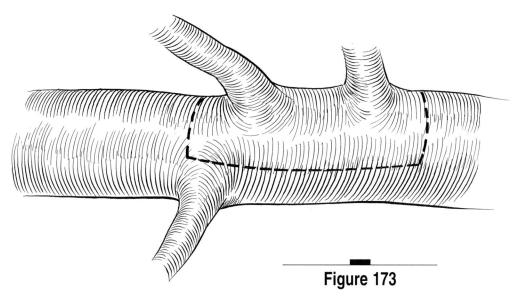

**Figure 173**

A rectangular aortotomy is created, allowing visualization of the visceral and renal ostia.

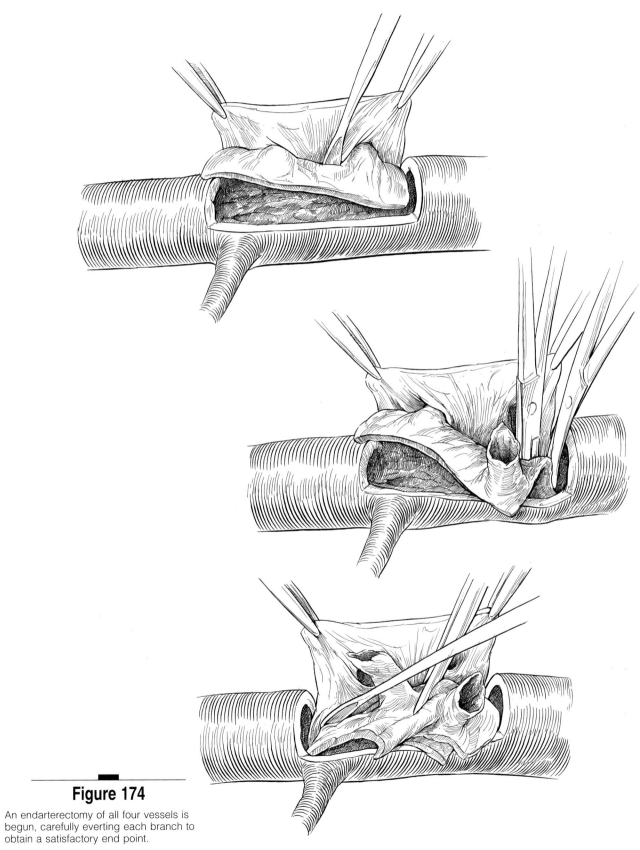

**Figure 174**

An endarterectomy of all four vessels is begun, carefully everting each branch to obtain a satisfactory end point.

### Mesenteric Arterial Bypass

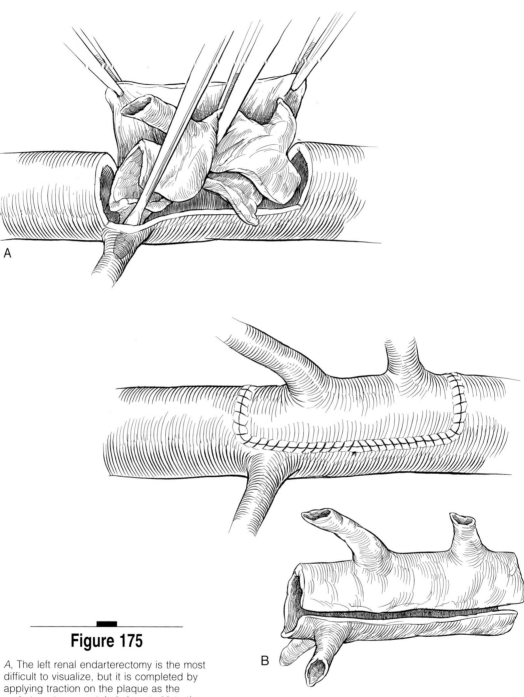

**Figure 175**

A, The left renal endarterectomy is the most difficult to visualize, but it is completed by applying traction on the plaque as the endarterectomy spatula is inserted into the proper plane in the left renal artery. B, The aortotomy is closed after removal of the plaque, which is occasionally delivered in one intact piece.

# CHAPTER 24

# Superior Mesenteric Artery Embolectomy

Mesenteric ischemia is appropriately divided into acute and chronic varieties. There is, however, some overlap between the two, as when an unrecognized mesenteric artery stenosis progresses to occlusion. Although chronic atherosclerotic occlusive disease of the superior mesenteric artery (SMA) alone is only occasionally associated with progression to thrombosis and development of acute ischemia (an entity that normally requires multivessel involvement), acute embolic occlusion of the SMA alone almost always results in intestinal infarction and rapid demise. Prompt diagnosis and aggressive treatment are essential before deterioration becomes irreversible.

In the classic form of acute mesenteric ischemia, the SMA is occluded by an embolus, usually of cardiac origin. The embolus generally lodges beyond the first few centimeters of the SMA, preserving flow through the proximal jejunal branches. This accounts for the characteristic findings at laparotomy of a spared proximal jejunum, in sharp contrast to SMA thrombosis, in which the process involves the SMA to its origin and occludes the proximal jejunal branches. Despite preformed collaterals, this process results in ischemia of the entire small intestine.

Embolism can be differentiated from thrombosis by a preoperative arteriogram. In cases of embolization, the anteroposterior arteriographic view usually demonstrates contrast filling of the first several centimeters of SMA, with a sharp cutoff and a meniscus occluding the vessel thereafter. Filling of the proximal jejunal branches is seen. In SMA thrombosis, however, the SMA is not visualized on the anteroposterior view, although a lateral view occasionally reveals a tapering stump of the vessel. The distinction between SMA embolism and thrombosis is important, because therapy for an embolus is embolectomy alone, whereas SMA thrombosis requires bypass of the occluded site.

*Superior Mesenteric Artery Embolectomy*

## OPERATIVE PROCEDURE

Embolectomy of the SMA is accomplished with exposure of the proximal portion of the SMA. Generally, a midline laparotomy is made, which affords adequate exposure for a thorough abdominal exploration, arterial reconstruction, and if necessary, bowel resection. The transverse colon is reflected cranially, and the SMA is palpated proximally in the mesentery. With this as a guide, the vessel is exposed as it crosses the duodenum (Fig. 176). A pulseless, rubbery vessel is consistent with embolization, and a firm, nodular, calcified vessel implies thrombosis of a chronic lesion. This condition and the extent of jejunal ischemia confirm the diagnosis.

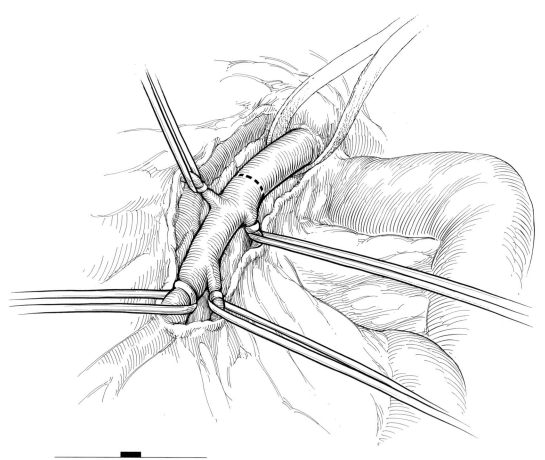

### Figure 176

Exposure of the superior mesenteric artery in the root of the mesentery as it crosses over the junction of the third and fourth portions of the duodenum.

The second segment of the SMA, near the middle colic branch, is exposed over a distance of several centimeters. The artery and its proximal branches are controlled with vessel loops. As with performance of any thromboembolectomy, it is unnecessary to tighten the vessel loops, because this action is likely to disrupt the thrombus. A transverse arteriotomy is made. A No. 4 balloon embolectomy catheter is passed proximally to retrieve thrombus and reestablish adequate inflow (Fig. 177). A smaller catheter, usually a No. 3, is then passed into the major superior mesenteric arterial branches (Fig. 178). The catheter is withdrawn, extruding the distal thrombus (Fig. 179). Additional thrombus may be removed from the smaller branches by milking the branches digitally and extruding the thrombus through the arteriotomy (Fig. 180).

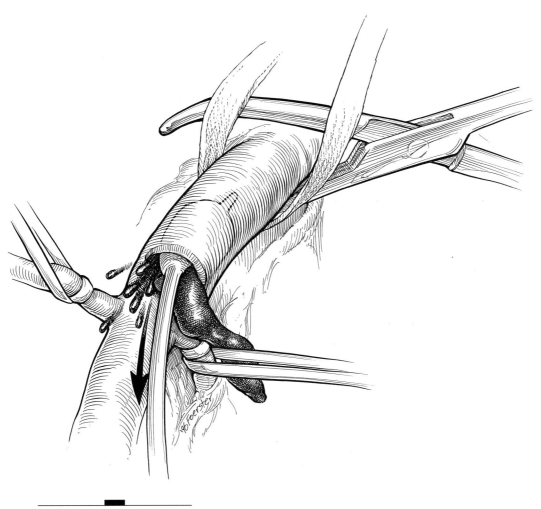

## Figure 177

A proximal thromboembolectomy, performed with a No. 4 balloon catheter.

*Superior Mesenteric Artery Embolectomy*

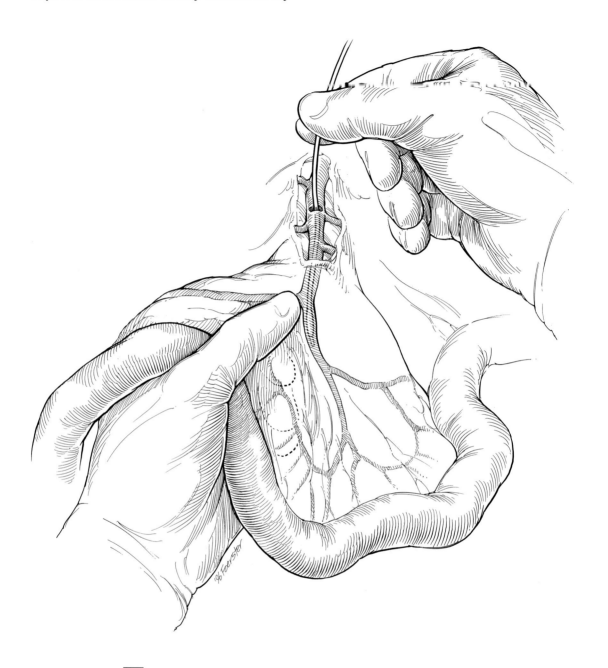

---

**Figure 178**

Distal thrombectomy of the superior
mesenteric artery and its branches.
Cannulation of individual branches is aided
with digital compression.

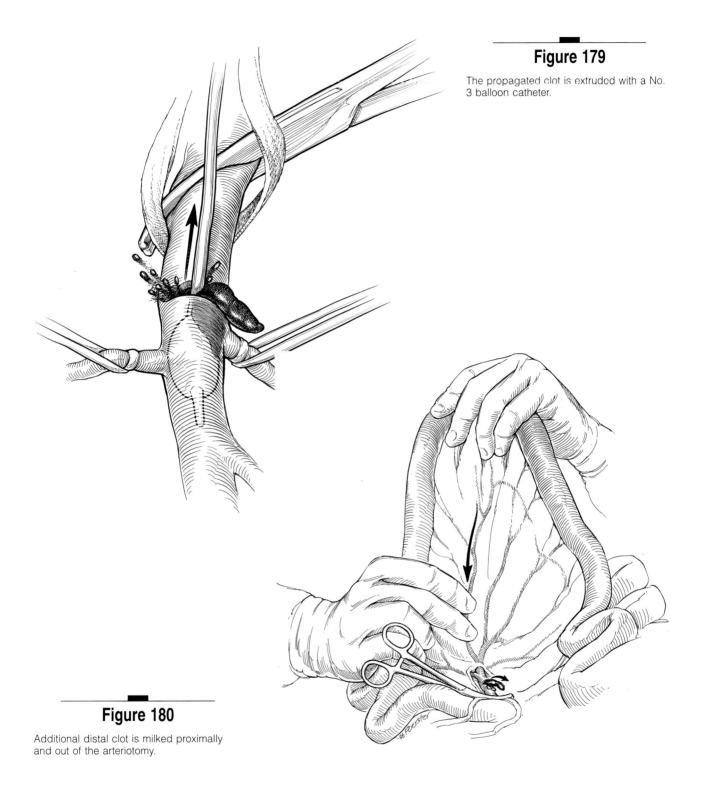

**Figure 179**

The propagated clot is extruded with a No. 3 balloon catheter.

**Figure 180**

Additional distal clot is milked proximally and out of the arteriotomy.

## Superior Mesenteric Artery Embolectomy

On completion of the embolectomy, the transverse arteriotomy is closed using interrupted 6-0 polypropylene sutures. Patency of the reconstruction is confirmed, using intraoperative Doppler or duplex ultrasonography.

Even after a successful thromboembolectomy, an ischemic portion of small or large intestine may remain (Fig. 181). Margins of viability are determined by inspection and contractility, and the determination is aided by eliciting audible Doppler arterial signals. Resection is frequently necessary, using primary anastomosis and second-look laparotomy (Fig. 182) or exteriorization (Fig. 183). This decision is made with consideration of the patient's condition and the need to conserve as much "marginal" intestine as possible. Although exteriorization is quickest and safest, subsequent restoration of bowel continuity may require sacrifice of additional bowel. Continued metabolic derangements are common despite an appropriate operation, accounting for an extremely high mortality rate after SMA embolization.

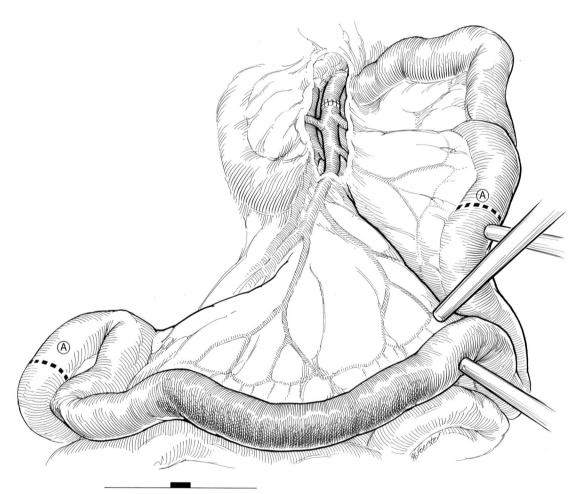

## Figure 181

Despite a technically adequate procedure, intestinal ischemia may persist, mandating resection.

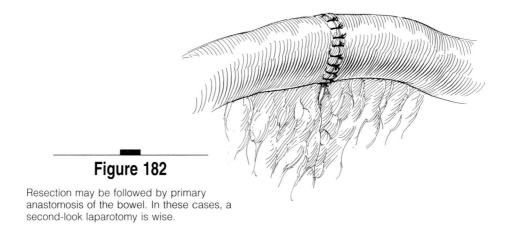

## Figure 182

Resection may be followed by primary
anastomosis of the bowel. In these cases, a
second-look laparotomy is wise.

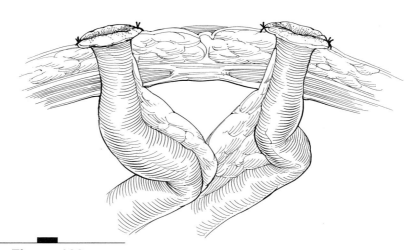

## Figure 183

As an alternative, sometimes safer
technique, the infarcted bowel can be
resected and the proximal and distal ends
exteriorized as enterostomies. This
approach affords the opportunity to easily
assess the viability of the remaining bowel.

# BRACHIOENCEPHALIC RECONSTRUCTION

# CHAPTER 25

# Carotid Endarterectomy

Carotid endarterectomy is the most frequently performed peripheral vascular surgical procedure in many practices. A decline in the number of carotid endarterectomies occurred during the late 1980s and early 1990s as a result of claimed improvements in medical therapy, such as antiplatelet agents and control of risk factors. This relative trend was reversed after the publication of several randomized trials comparing surgical with medical therapy for carotid disease, repudiating the effectiveness of medical therapy for severe carotid stenoses.

## OPERATIVE PROCEDURE

The neck is hyperextended with the chin turned away from the operative side (Fig. 184). A longitudinal incision is made along the anterior border of the sternocleidomastoid muscle. Some surgeons prefer a curvilinear incision running in a skin crease obliquely down and toward the midline, but we appreciate the ease with which the longitudinal incision may be extended proximally and distally when unsuspected common or distal internal carotid disease must be addressed.

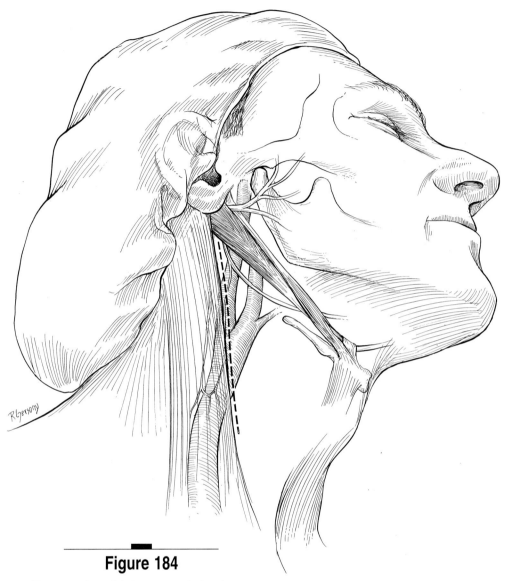

## Figure 184

The patient's neck is hyperextended and
turned away from the operative field in
preparation for a carotid endarterectomy. The
incision runs parallel to the anterior border of
the sternocleidomastoid muscle, along its
upper two thirds.

## Carotid Endarterectomy

The subcutaneous fat and platysma muscle are divided with electrocautery, ligating and dividing branches of the external jugular system running immediately beneath the platysmal layer. Dissection is continued in the plane around the anterior border of the sternocleidomastoid muscle. Lateral retraction of the muscle and continued medial dissection exposes the internal jugular vein. Its large facial tributary is ligated and divided along with a higher tributary running just superficial to the hypoglossal nerve. Division of these branches of the internal jugular vein allows the vein to be mobilized laterally, exposing the carotid bifurcation and the vagus nerve (Fig. 185).

The hypoglossal nerve is visualized as it crosses the internal and external carotid arteries; it is tethered inferiorly by a small artery running from the occipital artery to the sternocleidomastoid muscle. The ansa cervicalis also pulls the hypoglossal nerve inferiorly, and division of the ansa and the artery to the sternocleidomastoid muscle allows the hypoglossal nerve to be released medially as the first step in exposing the high internal carotid artery. The posterior belly of the digastric muscle may also be divided to obtain an additional 1 to 2 cm of distal exposure. Using these techniques, we have needed to subluxate the mandible only infrequently to gain high enough exposure.

After adequate heparinization, the external carotid artery is controlled with a vessel loop, and the superior thyroid artery is temporarily clipped. The internal carotid artery is occluded with a *gentle* bulldog clamp (e.g., Gregory) or surrounded with a vessel loop if an intraluminal shunt will be used. The proximal common carotid artery is controlled with a vessel loop and a vascular clamp.

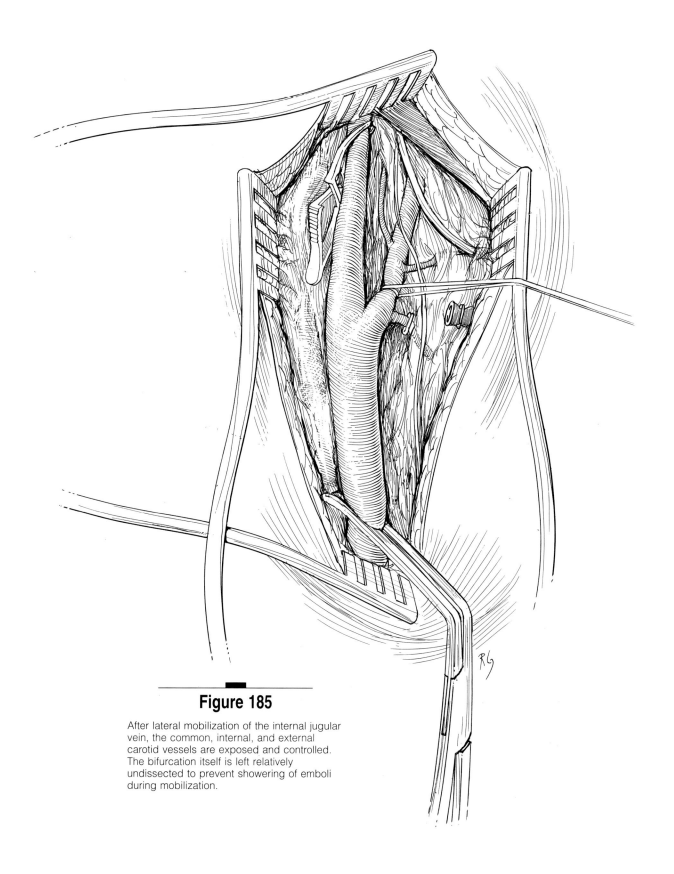

**Figure 185**

After lateral mobilization of the internal jugular
vein, the common, internal, and external
carotid vessels are exposed and controlled.
The bifurcation itself is left relatively
undissected to prevent showering of emboli
during mobilization.

## Carotid Endarterectomy

If desired, carotid stump pressures can be obtained at this time by inserting a "transduced" 23-gauge needle into the common carotid artery and momentarily releasing the internal carotid artery clamp. The absence of flow converts the internal carotid artery into a "manometer," reflecting the pressure at the circle of Willis. We have used a threshold mean stump pressure of 40 mm Hg to guide the need for shunting. If intraoperative electroencephalography is used instead, the tracing is observed for slowing, a sign that is usually manifested within 30 seconds of cross-clamping.

The carotid arteriotomy is begun on the common carotid artery, just proximal to palpable disease. The arteriotomy is continued distally, skirting the external carotid orifice, to end on healthy internal carotid vessel. When deemed necessary, the surgeon places a shunt at this time, inserting the internal carotid end first and allowing backbleeding to evacuate air from the tube before inserting the common carotid end.

The endarterectomy is begun at the site of the heaviest plaque formation, because the plane is most easily developed at this point. A spatula is inserted beneath the plaque, developing the natural plane of separation between the plaque and the residual outer media and adventitia at the site of the external elastic lamella. The proximal end of the plaque is divided with the Potts scissors or with a No. 15 blade over the spatula, and the endarterectomy is carried distally with longitudinal motions of the spatula to elevate the plaque off the residual arterial wall (Fig. 186). The external carotid artery loop is briefly released to allow an eversion endarterectomy of this vessel.

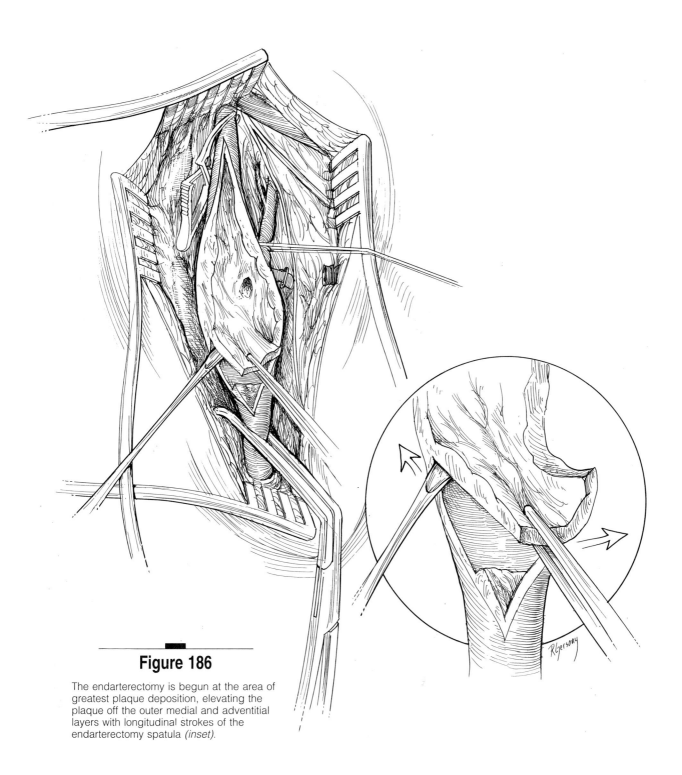

## Figure 186

The endarterectomy is begun at the area of greatest plaque deposition, elevating the plaque off the outer medial and adventitial layers with longitudinal strokes of the endarterectomy spatula *(inset)*.

## Carotid Endarterectomy

The plaque is elevated off the internal carotid artery, while the surgeon pays particular attention to the transition zone where the plaque becomes thinner and localized to the intimal layer. The media is normal at this point and is adherent to the adventitia. A transverse line between the reddish adventitia and the white medial layers is readily visualized. Often, the plaque separates cleanly with traction alone; otherwise, lateral traction on the plaque, sometimes assisted by making a nick with fine Potts or iris scissors, allows the plaque to peel away and leave a second transition zone from the adherent media to the thin, translucent intima (Fig. 187). The endarterectomized surface is cleared of residual circular medial fibers, removing them with a fine forceps and heparinized saline irrigation.

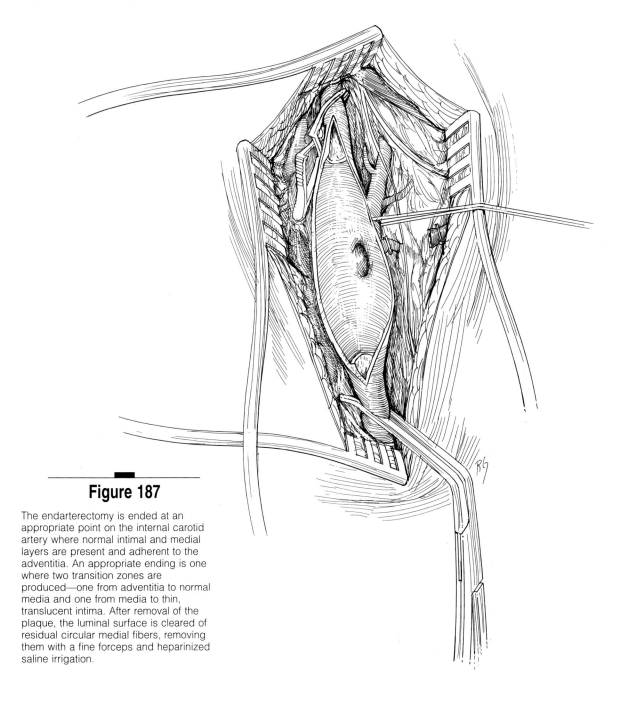

### Figure 187

The endarterectomy is ended at an appropriate point on the internal carotid artery where normal intimal and medial layers are present and adherent to the adventitia. An appropriate ending is one where two transition zones are produced—one from adventitia to normal media and one from media to thin, translucent intima. After removal of the plaque, the luminal surface is cleared of residual circular medial fibers, removing them with a fine forceps and heparinized saline irrigation.

The arteriotomy is closed primarily or with a patch (Fig. 188). It has been our practice to patch all but the largest internal carotid arteries with a single, running 6-0 polypropylene suture and fashioned, precut coated polyester material. Some surgeons have used saphenous vein patches, and others have used everted, doubled external jugular vein. The patch is intended to restore the appropriate luminal dimension without enlarging it significantly.

If a shunt has been employed, it is removed before placement of the last few sutures. Air and debris are flushed out of the bifurcation before release of the distal clamp; the internal carotid clamp is released last.

The technical result is assessed with Doppler ultrasonography, a duplex ultrasound probe, or arteriography. Protamine sulfate reversal of the heparin effects and wound drainage are used at the surgeon's discretion. If desired, a drain is placed through a stab wound low in the neck. The drain may be removed after the heparin has worn off, usually within 6 hours. The platysma is closed with a running absorbable suture, and the skin is closed with a subcuticular stitch. Postoperative carotid surveillance is performed with duplex ultrasonography before discharge and at 6-month intervals for the first 2 postoperative years.

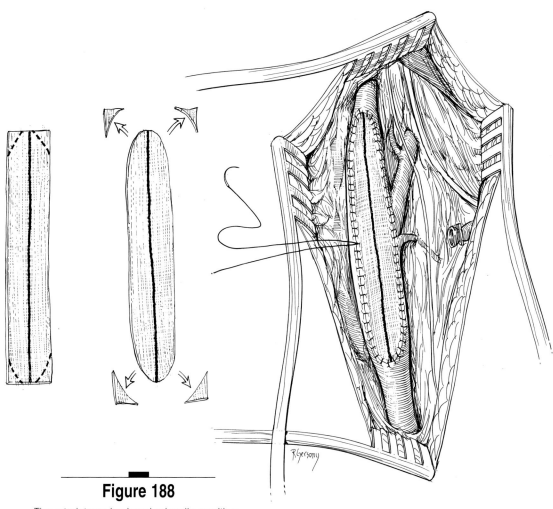

## Figure 188

The arteriotomy is closed primarily or with a patch. Polyester carotid patch material may be precut or may require fashioning of the ends to achieve an appropriate shape.

# CHAPTER 26

# Subclavian to Carotid Transposition

A subclavian to carotid transposition is performed in the setting of proximal subclavian arterial occlusion, most commonly for subclavian steal syndrome. A normal proximal common carotid artery is a prerequisite, and the subclavian disease must terminate well proximal to the vertebral origin. The procedure is performed only in symptomatic patients. Asymptomatic subclavian steal is not an indication for a subclavian arterial reconstruction. Candidates must manifest symptoms of vertebrobasilar hypoperfusion, vertebrobasilar embolization, severely symptomatic upper extremity ischemia, or digital embolization.

The first group of patients includes those who have vertebrobasilar symptoms because of posterior cerebral hypoperfusion or, occasionally, embolization through the vertebral arteries. A severely stenotic subclavian lesion is never the source of posterior circulation emboli, because the flow in the vertebral artery is retrograde in these cases, precluding embolization to the brain. However, posterior cerebral hypoperfusion commonly occurs *only* in the presence of severe, hemodynamically significant subclavian disease. The candidate must have bilateral subclavian and vertebral disease or hypoplasia, because one normal vertebral artery is all that is necessary to maintain adequate posterior cerebral perfusion. Moreover, symptomatic posterior cerebral hypoperfusion does not occur unless there exists another lesion that interferes with compensatory collateral flow from the anterior cerebral (carotid) circulation. This lesion may be in the intracerebral communicating arteries (e.g., a diseased or absent posterior communicating artery) or in the carotid arteries themselves.

Severe, bilateral carotid disease is a frequent finding in patients with global symptoms. Unless the vertebrobasilar symptoms are thought to be embolic, such anterior lesions should be sought and repaired first. If carotid stenosis is hemodynamically significant (e.g., greater than 60% reduction in diameter), our experience suggests that classic vertebrobasilar insufficiency can be relieved in most cases. Unrestricted flow through the posterior communicating arteries in the circle of Willis usually can provide adequate posterior cerebral blood flow to ameliorate the symptoms. Subclavian or vertebral lesions should be addressed only when symptoms continue after correction of the carotid disease.

Rarely, a subclavian arterial reconstruction becomes necessary for upper extremity ischemic symptoms. The symptoms are often embolic, with evidence of digital ischemic changes or gangrene. Alternatively, the symptoms may be those of rest pain or severe upper extremity claudication. Severe claudication symptoms occur infrequently because of the abundant collateral flow around subclavian stenoses. This observation explains the discrepancy between the common finding of the arteriographic manifestation of subclavian steal and the infrequency of symptoms sufficient to warrant operative intervention. In patients with coronary artery bypass grafts in whom the internal mammary artery was used, subclavian stenoses may result in recurrent angina and require repair.

When subclavian arterial reconstruction is needed, a subclavian to carotid transposition offers advantages over the more frequently performed carotid to subclavian bypass. A subclavian to carotid transposition does not involve the use of a bypass conduit, only one anastomosis is required, and the subclavian lesion is excluded from the circulation, obviating the risk of embolization.

## OPERATIVE PROCEDURE

The common carotid and subclavian arteries are exposed through a transverse supraclavicular approach. The patient's neck is hyperextended, with the head turned away and the shoulder depressed, to bring the subclavian artery out from beneath the clavicle. The supraclavicular region is sterilely prepared, as is the anterior chest.

An incision is made approximately 1 to 2 cm superior to the clavicle, running laterally from the lateral edge of the sternal head of the sternocleidomastoid muscle for a distance of approximately 10 cm (Fig. 189). The platysma is divided with electrocautery, as is the clavicular head of the sternocleidomastoid and the omohyoid muscle (Fig. 190). The scalene fat pad, with its abundant lymphatics, small arteries, and veins, is ligated in continuity, divided along its inferior and lateral margins, and reflected cephalad. The anterior scalene muscle is visualized, with the phrenic nerve coursing inferiorly across its muscle fibers (Fig. 191). The muscle is divided, with the phrenic nerve being carefully protected in the process (Fig. 192). Throughout the exposure, care is taken to avoid the area of the thoracic duct, which is encountered as it loops anteriorly to enter the superolateral junction of the left subclavian and internal jugular veins.

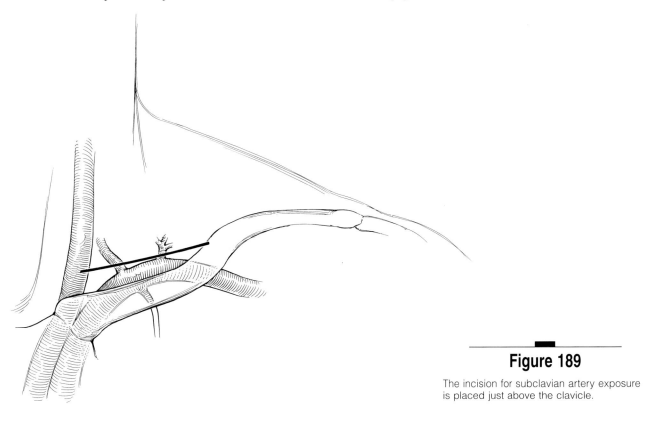

**Figure 189**

The incision for subclavian artery exposure is placed just above the clavicle.

**Subclavian to Carotid Transposition**

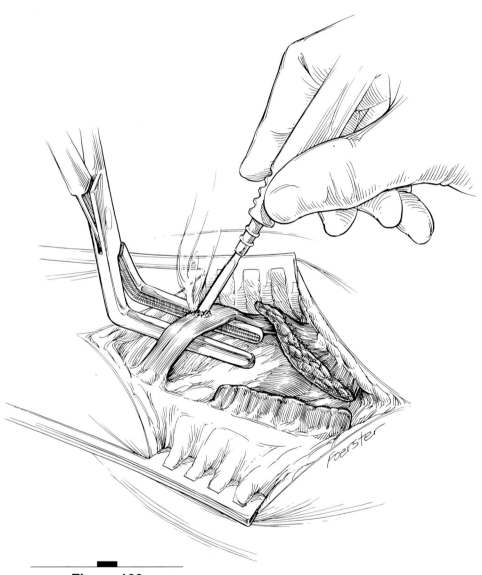

## Figure 190

After division of the platysma and the lateral head of the sternocleidomastoid muscle, the omohyoid is divided with electrocautery.

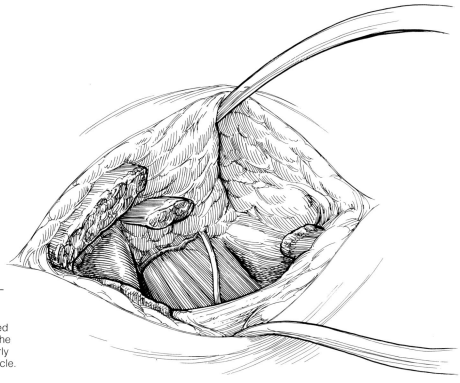

## Figure 191

The anterior scalene muscle is exposed after division of the scalene fat pad. The phrenic nerve is seen coursing inferiorly across the anterior surface of the muscle.

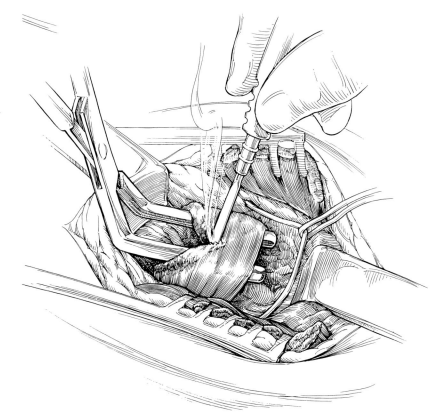

## Figure 192

The anterior scalene muscle is divided while care is taken to protect the phrenic nerve. The subclavian artery lies immediately deep to the inferior portion of the muscle.

## *Subclavian to Carotid Transposition*

The subclavian artery is found immediately deep to the anterior scalene muscle. Just as division of the pectoralis minor muscle is the gateway to the axillary artery, so is the anterior scalene muscle the key to exposure of the subclavian artery. Once identified, the fragile artery is gently cleared of surrounding tissue (Fig. 193), with ligation and division of the thyrocervical and costocervical trunks as necessary. Unlike other supraclavicular procedures, a transposition requires additional medial exposure of the proximal subclavian artery well below the origin of the vertebral artery. The vertebral artery is identified as exiting the subclavian artery on its posterosuperior aspect (Fig. 194). The subclavian artery is mobilized as far proximally as possible, well into the mediastinum.

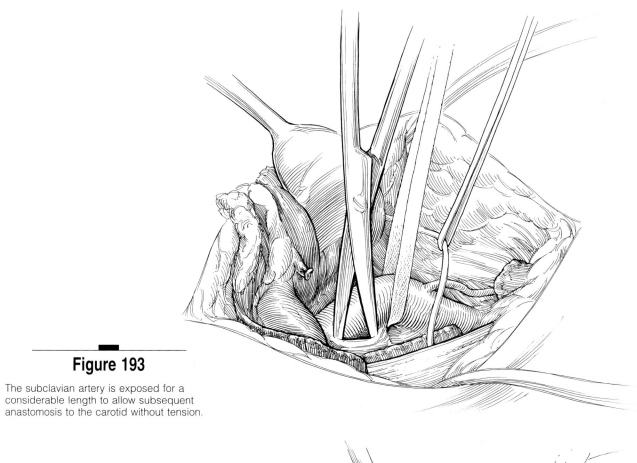

## Figure 193

The subclavian artery is exposed for a considerable length to allow subsequent anastomosis to the carotid without tension.

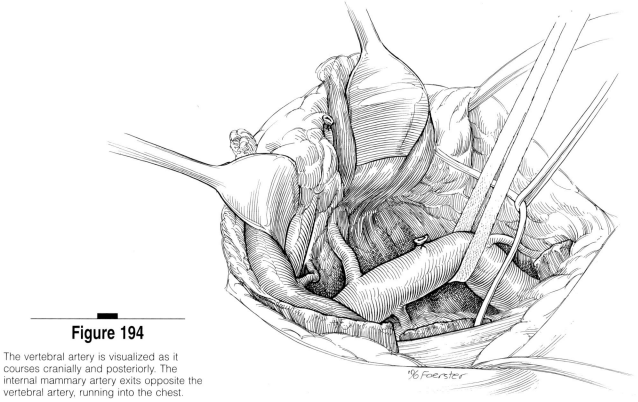

## Figure 194

The vertebral artery is visualized as it courses cranially and posteriorly. The internal mammary artery exits opposite the vertebral artery, running into the chest.

## Subclavian to Carotid Transposition

The common carotid artery is exposed with medial retraction of the internal jugular vein while avoiding injury to the vagus nerve lying in the groove between the artery and the vein (Fig. 195). Mobilization of the pliable common carotid artery over a substantial distance allows the vessel to be more easily juxtaposed to the subclavian artery. In many cases, the internal mammary artery must be divided to allow the subclavian artery to reach the common carotid artery. This potential drawback must always be considered in patients with known or suspected coronary artery disease. Mobilization of the vertebral artery over 1 to 2 cm allows the subclavian artery to rotate cranially for anastomosis (Fig. 196).

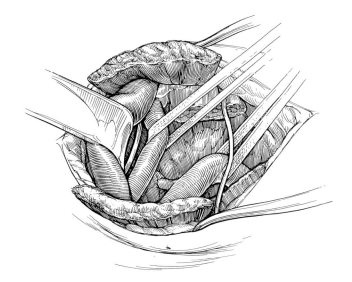

## Figure 195

Through the same incision, the common carotid artery is exposed. The vessel is found beneath the internal jugular vein, with the vagus nerve lying in the groove between the artery and vein.

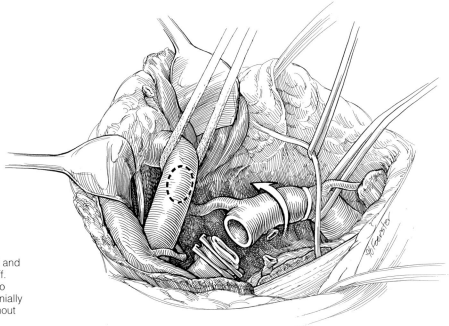

## Figure 196

The subclavian artery is doubly clipped and divided proximal to the vertebral take-off. Adequate vertebral artery is mobilized to allow the subclavian artery to rotate cranially to reach the common carotid artery without kinking.

## *Subclavian to Carotid Transposition*

After heparinization, the proximal subclavian artery is divided between clamps, and the proximal stump is ligated with polypropylene suture or doubly clipped. An ellipse of arterial wall is excised from the common carotid vessel, and the subclavian artery is rotated 90° to prevent kinking of the vertebral artery. The end-to-side anastomosis is begun in the posterior midline with 5-0 or 6-0 polypropylene suture in a running fashion (Fig. 197). On release of the clamps, care is taken to prevent air or debris from traveling distally through the common carotid circulation or the vertebral artery. The distal common carotid and vertebral clamps are removed last (Fig. 198).

The wound is closed with running absorbable suture for the platysmal layer and running subcuticular suture for the skin. A drain is used, especially when the procedure has been performed on the left side, and it is removed on the second or third postoperative day, after the absence of lymphatic leakage has been confirmed.

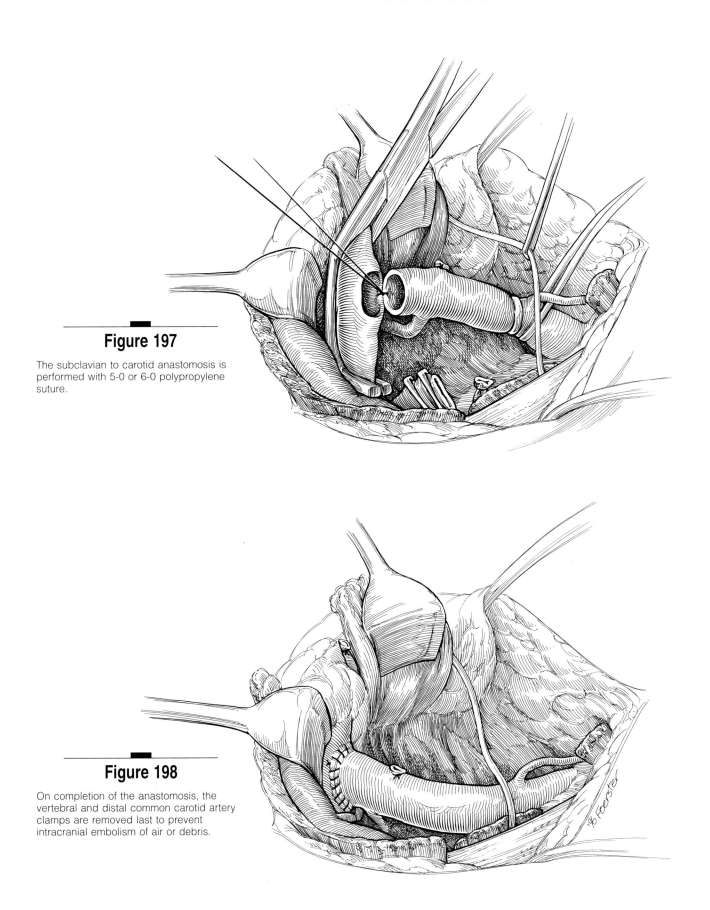

**Figure 197**

The subclavian to carotid anastomosis is performed with 5-0 or 6-0 polypropylene suture.

**Figure 198**

On completion of the anastomosis, the vertebral and distal common carotid artery clamps are removed last to prevent intracranial embolism of air or debris.

# CHAPTER 27

# Carotid to Subclavian Transposition

A carotid to subclavian transposition is the procedure of choice for isolated proximal common carotid disease. The procedure is easier than a subclavian to carotid transposition from a technical standpoint, because the procurement of a long length of common carotid artery is relatively straightforward. Unfortunately, coexistent proximal subclavian disease may contraindicate the use of this procedure. Nevertheless, when the proximal subclavian artery is free of stenosis, the carotid to subclavian bypass provides an attractive extrathoracic means of restoring normal flow to the common carotid artery with a single anastomosis and without the use of a prosthetic conduit.

## OPERATIVE PROCEDURE

The operation is begun with the standard supraclavicular exposure of the subclavian artery and performed under general anesthesia with the head hyperextended and turned away from the operative side. The lateral head of the sternocleidomastoid muscle is divided, as is the scalene fat pad. The phrenic nerve is identified, and the anterior scalene muscle is divided. A suitable length of subclavian artery is exposed, ligating the thyrocervical and costocervical trunks as necessary (Fig. 199). Care must be exercised to leave the vertebral and internal mammary arteries undisturbed.

The common carotid artery is exposed by retracting the remaining portion of the sternocleidomastoid muscle and the internal jugular vein medially (Fig. 200). The vagus nerve is usually visualized during this maneuver, and care is taken to leave the nerve undisturbed. Occasionally, the initial exposure of the common carotid artery may be more easily achieved by retracting the internal jugular vein laterally. In this case, after the artery has been identified, it is slipped deep to the jugular vein in preparation for more proximal exposure, division, and anastomosis. A long length of common carotid artery is mobilized well into the mediastinum to allow easy anastomosis to the subclavian vessel. The area of the thoracic duct is avoided when operating on theleft side, keeping the dissection away from the junction of the internal jugular and subclavian veins.

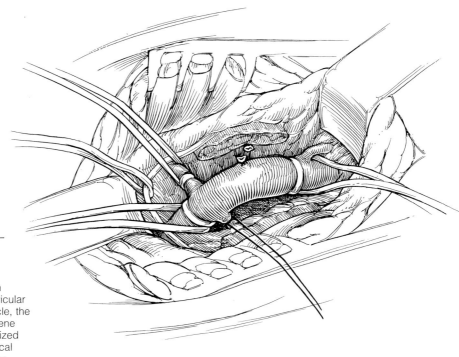

## Figure 199

Exposure of the subclavian artery in preparation for a carotid to subclavian transposition. After division of the clavicular head of the sternocleidomastoid muscle, the scalene fat pad, and the anterior scalene muscle, the subclavian artery is mobilized and controlled, dividing the thyrocervical and costocervical trunks, as necessary.

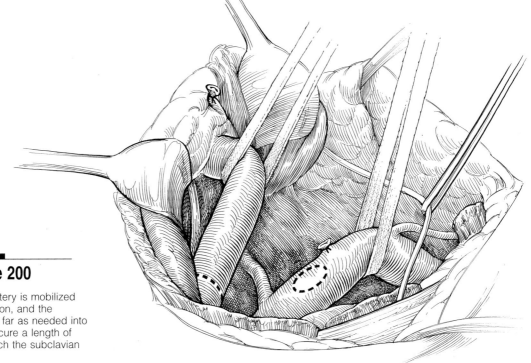

## Figure 200

The common carotid artery is mobilized through the same incision, and the dissection is carried as far as needed into the mediastinum to procure a length of vessel adequate to reach the subclavian

## Carotid to Subclavian Transposition

After heparinization, the most proximal common carotid artery is clamped and divided, and the proximal stump is oversewn with polypropylene suture. A subclavian arteriotomy is made linearly or in an elliptical fashion. An end-to-side anastomosis is then constructed (Fig. 201) with 5-0 or 6-0 polypropylene suture. It is almost never necessary to employ an indwelling shunt during performance of this anastomosis, because clamping of the common carotid artery is usually well tolerated, especially in the presence of long-standing proximal stenosis.

The clamps are released on completion of the anastomosis, with the distal carotid clamp being removed last to prevent cerebral embolization (Fig. 202). The patency of the reconstruction is established with digital palpation, Doppler, or intraoperative duplex ultrasonography. After placement of a drain, the incision is closed using absorbable suture for the platysma layer and a subcuticular running suture or clips for the skin. The drain is removed on the first or second postoperative day unless lymphatic drainage indicative of an injury to the thoracic duct is discovered.

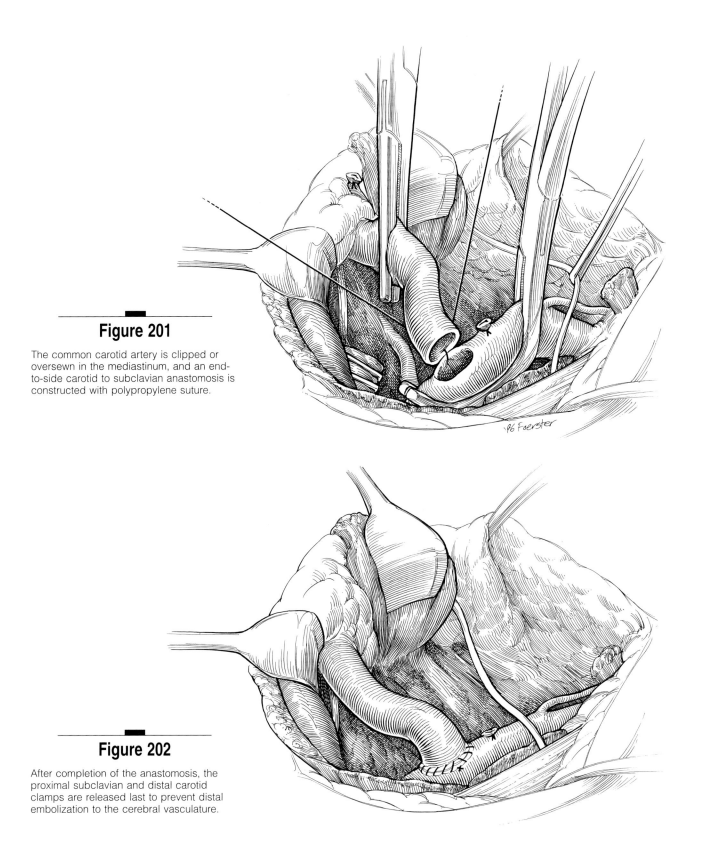

**Figure 201**

The common carotid artery is clipped or oversewn in the mediastinum, and an end-to-side carotid to subclavian anastomosis is constructed with polypropylene suture.

**Figure 202**

After completion of the anastomosis, the proximal subclavian and distal carotid clamps are released last to prevent distal embolization to the cerebral vasculature.

# CHAPTER 28

# Carotid to Subclavian Bypass

A carotid to subclavian bypass may be performed in the setting of vessel proximal subclavian or proximal common carotid disease. It can be considered a rival of the carotid to subclavian transpositions described in previous chapters. The indications for the operation are identical to those described in Chapters 26 and 27. Because of this versatility, the procedure has become the most commonly performed operation for proximal brachiocephalic disease. If the preoperative indications are those of embolization, the procedure must be combined with proximal ligation or end-to-end distal anastomosis to exclude the embolic source. In general, prosthetic grafts (i.e., ePTFE or polyester) are preferred instead of saphenous vein because of the presumed inferior patency rates with an autogenous graft, possibly related to graft kinking during flexion of the neck. For this reason, externally supported (i.e., ringed) prostheses are employed.

## OPERATIVE PROCEDURE

The procedure is carried out through a standard supraclavicular approach to the subclavian and common carotid vessels. The subclavian artery need not be exposed as far proximally as is necessary with a subclavian to carotid transposition, because the anastomosis is performed at its apex. This aspect of the subclavian artery and its branches are controlled, the patient is administered heparin, and the vessels are clamped.

The anastomosis to the prosthetic graft is constructed on the anterosuperior aspect of the subclavian artery (Fig. 203). It is critical to choose the correct length of graft to avoid tension or kinking. With one anastomosis completed, the neck can be moved back toward a more neutral position to allow the appropriate length to be determined with confidence.

A common carotid arteriotomy is made on the lateral wall of the vessel, excising an ellipse to improve the contour and ease of sewing the anastomosis (Fig. 204). The anastomosis is then constructed with running 5-0 or 6-0 suture. The occluding clamps are removed after completion of the anastomosis, releasing the distal common carotid and vertebral clamps last to prevent cerebral embolization.

On completion of the anastomoses, the graft makes a gentle arc in the supraclavicular fossa. The wound is closed over a drain, using running absorbable suture for the platysmal layer and clips or subcuticular suture for the skin.

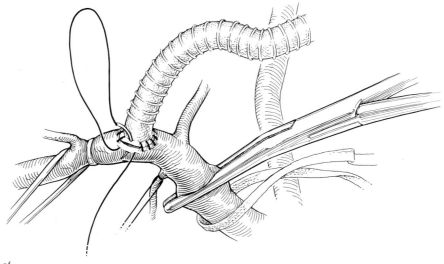

## Figure 203

After a standard supraclavicular exposure of the subclavian and common carotid arteries, the subclavian artery is clamped, and an end-to-side anastomosis is constructed. An externally supported ePTFE graft is depicted.

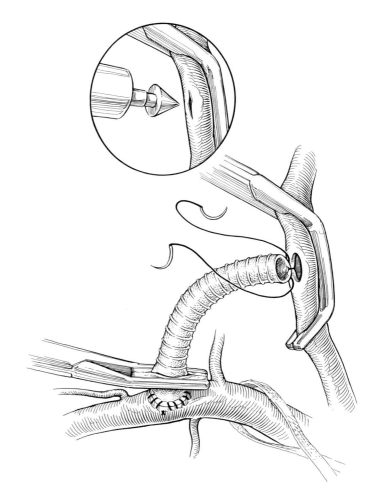

## Figure 204

The carotid arteriotomy is made with a hole punch *(inset)*, facilitating construction of the end-to-side anastomosis. On completion of the anastomosis, the externally supported graft makes a gentle arc in the supraclavicular fossa, discouraging kinking during cervical flexion.

# CHAPTER 29

# Subclavian to Carotid Bypass With Carotid Bifurcation Endarterectomy

A subclavian to carotid bypass is necessary for treating tandem disease of the proximal common carotid artery and the carotid bifurcation. The bifurcation disease may be picked up by duplex ultrasonography, which may miss intrathoracic common carotid lesions. For this reason, the supraclavicular region must be prepared when performing a carotid endarterectomy without preoperative arteriography. The surgeon then can use the subclavian artery for inflow if an abnormal common carotid pulse is detected. Occasionally, the subclavian to carotid bypass can be used in place of a carotid to subclavian transposition if the common carotid is diffusely diseased.

## OPERATIVE PROCEDURE

The operation is performed through two incisions: a longitudinal incision at the medial border of the sternocleidomastoid muscle and a transverse incision parallel to the clavicle. The procedure is begun with the normal exposure of the carotid bifurcation, retracting the internal jugular vein laterally and surrounding the internal, external, and common carotid vessels with vessel loops (Fig. 205). The subclavian artery is then exposed through the supraclavicular incision, transecting the clavicular head of the sternocleidomastoid muscle and the anterior scalene muscle and carefully retracting the phrenic nerve out of harm's way. A tunnel is bluntly developed between the two incisions (Fig. 206), and preparation is made for performance of the proximal anastomosis.

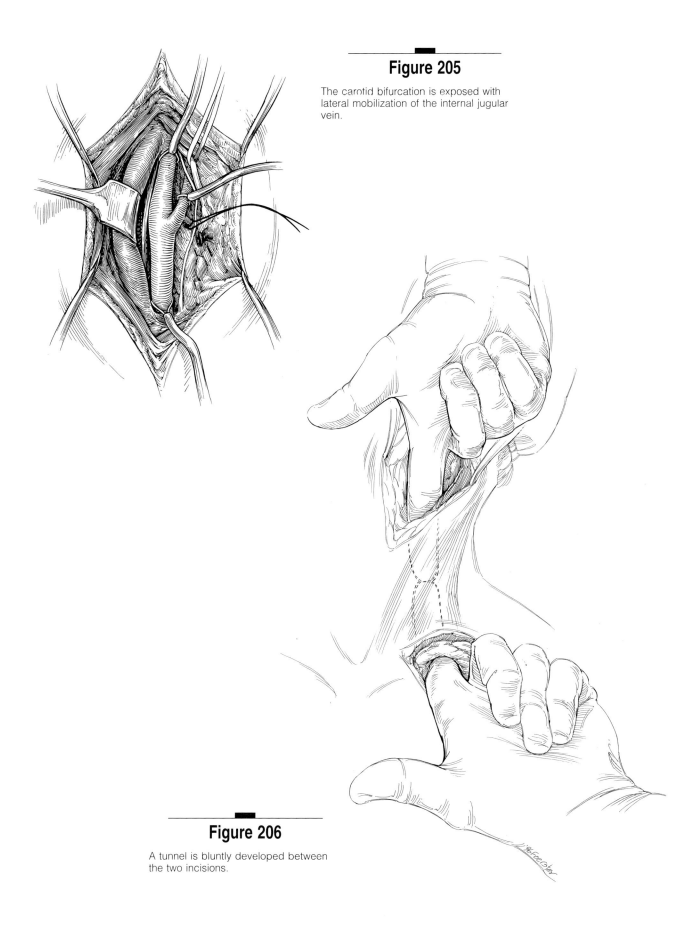

**Figure 205**

The carotid bifurcation is exposed with lateral mobilization of the internal jugular vein.

**Figure 206**

A tunnel is bluntly developed between the two incisions.

## Subclavian to Carotid Bypass With Carotid Bifurcation Endarterectomy

The patient is administered heparin, the subclavian artery is clamped proximally and distally, and an end-to-side anastomosis is constructed. A polyester or ePTFE graft may be used, and the anastomosis is sewn with 5-0 or 6-0 polypropylene suture. We prefer to use an externally supported ePTFE graft to avoid kinking with flexion or rotation of the neck. The graft is brought through the subcutaneous tunnel on completion of the anastomosis (Fig. 207).

The carotid vessels are clamped, and an endarterectomy is performed in the standard fashion. The bypass graft is then sewn to the arteriotomy, with the graft itself acting as a patch angioplasty for closure. Fine (6-0) polypropylene suture typically is used for this anastomosis (Fig. 208). The air and debris are flushed from the graft before release of the internal carotid clamp, and heparin is reversed with protamine sulfate after Doppler or duplex ultrasonography confirms the technical adequacy of the revascularization.

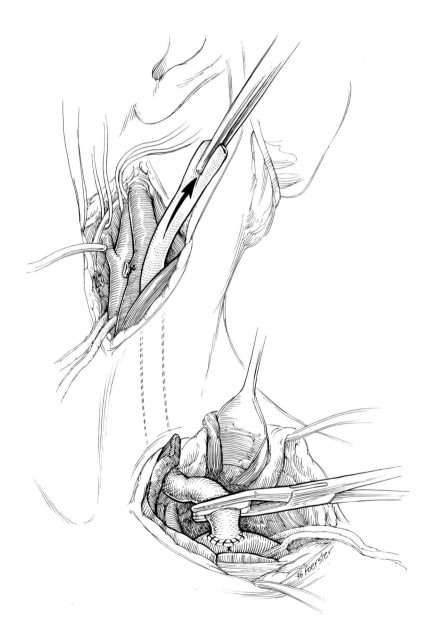

## Figure 207

The proximal anastomosis is performed in an end-to-side fashion, bringing the graft through the tunnel to the carotid bifurcation.

Performance of a distal end-to-side anastomosis is unwise when emboli from the proximal common carotid lesion are suspected. In these cases, the common carotid artery should be transected just proximal to the external carotid origin. The distal anastomosis of the subclavian to carotid bypass is then performed in an oblique end-to-end fashion, carefully tapering the hood of the graft over the internal carotid arteriotomy.

The wounds are closed using running suture for the platysmal layers and clips or absorbable subcuticular suture for the skin. A drain is used for the supraclavicular incision, especially when the procedure is performed in the left side of the neck. The drain is removed on the first or second postoperative day, once the absence of excessive lymphatic drainage has been confirmed.

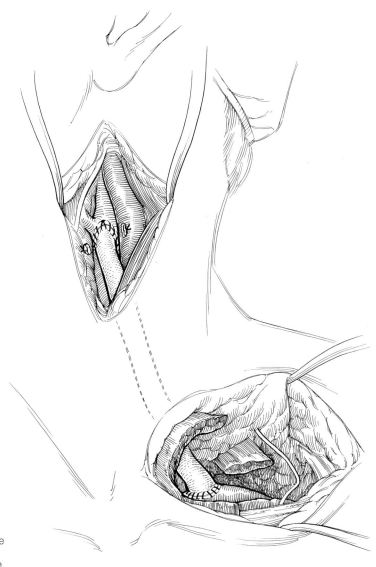

**Figure 208**

After a standard carotid endarterectomy, the graft is sewn over the carotid arteriotomy and functions as a patch closure at this site. If the proximal common carotid artery is suspected as the site of embolization, it should be excluded with proximal ligation or an end-to-end distal graft anastomosis.

# CHAPTER 30

# Carotid to Carotid Bypass

A carotid to carotid bypass is performed in the setting of proximal common carotid disease when the ipsilateral subclavian artery is diseased and is inappropriate as a source of inflow. The situation arises in cases of disease involving the aortic arch and its major branches, such as coexistent proximal common carotid and subclavian disease, or in some cases of innominate artery narrowing. A bifurcation endarterectomy may also be required in the face of tandem common and internal carotid disease.

The ascending aorta is the ideal inflow site in the bypass of multivessel brachiocephalic arterial occlusive disease. The carotid to carotid bypass is reserved for patients in whom a median sternotomy to obtain ascending aortic inflow is contraindicated by previous mediastinal surgery or compromised medical status.

## OPERATIVE PROCEDURE

The patient is placed in the supine position, with the neck hyperextended. This position allows two anterolateral incisions to be employed concurrently: a donor incision, running parallel to the lower two thirds of the medial border of the sternocleidomastoid muscle at the base of the neck, and a recipient incision, running parallel to the upper two thirds of the muscle to the angle of the mandible (Fig. 209).

The donor proximal common carotid artery is exposed by retracting the sternocleidomastoid muscle and internal jugular vein laterally. The recipient carotid vessel is exposed in the usual fashion for performing a carotid endarterectomy, which may be required in addition to the bypass. The polyester or ePTFE graft may be tunneled in an anterior subcutaneous position. We prefer to tunnel the graft through a retropharyngeal route, which permits a significantly shortened graft length and avoids an unsightly bulge in the neck of thin persons. A relatively small-diameter graft (6 mm) is adequate and obviates postoperative swallowing difficulties.

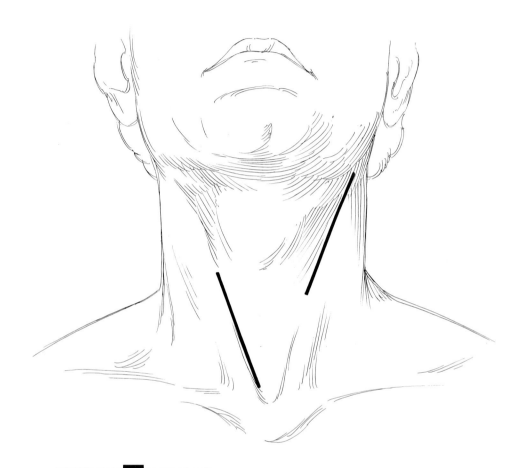

**Figure 209**

A carotid to carotid bypass is performed
through bilateral cervical incisions along
the medial border of each
sternocleidomastoid muscle. The
exposure on the inflow side is positioned
at the base of the neck, and the
contralateral incision is placed over the
carotid bifurcation.

## *Carotid to Carotid Bypass*

The patient is administered heparin, and clamps are applied to the donor carotid vessel. The need for a shunt at this point is rare, because temporary occlusion of the common carotid artery is infrequently associated with cerebral hypoperfusion, in contrast to the effect of clamping of the internal carotid artery.

The proximal anastomosis is completed in a beveled fashion with 5-0 or 6-0 polypropylene or comparable suture (Fig. 210). The recipient anastomosis is performed in a similar fashion. The distal carotid clamps are removed last to prevent embolization of air or debris. A shunt may be needed at this point if a concomitant carotid bifurcation endarterectomy is performed. The distal anastomosis may be done in an end-to-end fashion or with common carotid ligation if embolization from the proximal carotid lesion is suspected. The incisions are closed using absorbable suture for the platysma and clips or a running subcuticular suture for the skin.

Because of the bilateral exposures, adequacy of the patient's airway must be carefully monitored during the early postoperative period. Although rare, injury to both vagus nerves may result in airway obstruction from bilateral vocal chord paralysis. Alternatively, bilateral neck hematomas may quickly compromise the upper airway of patients with these transcervical grafts. For this reason, Silastic suction drains are left in place for the first several hours, until the effect of heparin has worn off and to ensure postoperative bleeding has not occurred.

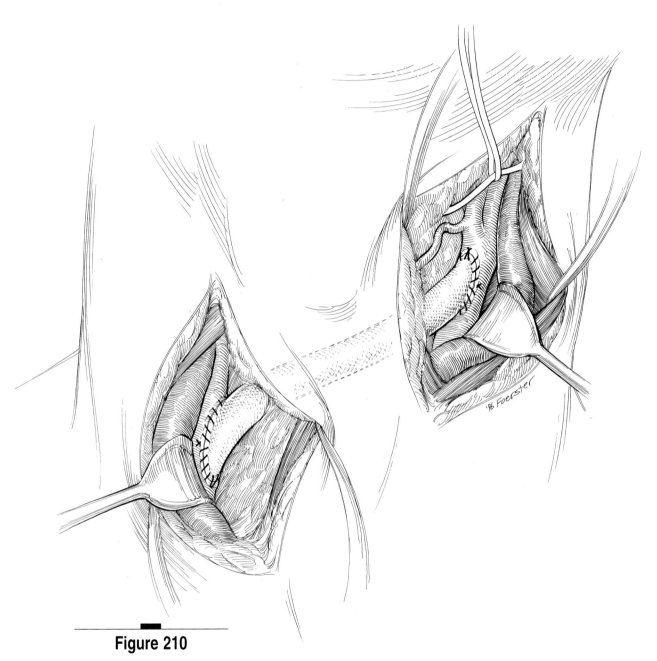

**Figure 210**

The completed carotid to carotid bypass graft has end-to-side anastomoses proximally and distally. The graft can be tunneled retropharyngeally to minimize the length of the graft and avoid an unsightly bulge on the anterior neck of thin persons. A carotid endarterectomy may be necessary at the site of the distal anastomosis. The distal anastomosis may be done in an end-to-end fashion or with common carotid ligation if embolization from the proximal carotid lesion is suspected.

# CHAPTER 31

# Vertebral to Carotid Transposition

A vertebral to carotid transposition is indicated for treating symptomatic proximal vertebral artery stenosis. Symptoms may occur as the result of embolization or, more commonly, posterior circulation hypoperfusion. Bilateral vertebral artery disease is necessary to produce such hypoperfusion, although symptoms occasionally develop with unilateral stenosis associated with an atrophic or congenitally absent contralateral vertebral artery. Less frequently, vertebral lesions may be the source of posterior circulation emboli, in which case vertebral reconstruction is necessary even though the contralateral vertebral vessel may be normal. The indications for vertebral artery transposition are limited, but when required, this procedure is preferred to others such as endarterectomy and patch angioplasty.

## OPERATIVE PROCEDURE

The vertebral artery is exposed through a supraclavicular incision, exposing the subclavian artery beneath the anterior scalene muscle and following the artery medially until the vertebral artery is identified (Fig. 211). The phrenic nerve is carefully protected to avoid temporary or permanent diaphragmatic paralysis, a problem that is poorly tolerated by patients with chronic lung disease. The thyrocervical trunk may be mistaken for the vertebral artery, but distal dissection quickly reveals the characteristic branching of the former.

The common carotid artery is exposed, along with anteromedial mobilization of the internal jugular vein. An adequate length of common carotid is freed proximally and distally. The vertebral artery is mobilized for a distance of 2 to 3 cm, taking care to avoid injury to the fragile vertebral vein.

After adequate heparinization, the vertebral artery is ligated proximally and transected. A side-biting clamp provides efficient control of the common carotid artery (Fig. 212), although the small size of the carotid precludes partial side clamping of the vessel as a means of preserving antegrade flow during construction of the anastomosis. Fortunately, unilateral common carotid occlusion is almost universally tolerated without the risk of cerebral infarction.

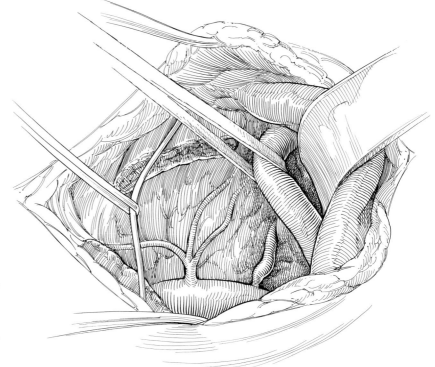

### Figure 211

Approach to the vertebral artery and the common carotid artery through a supraclavicular incision. The vertebral artery is exposed for a distance of several centimeters. If necessary, the vessel can be mobilized until it enters the foramen transversarium of the sixth cervical vertebra.

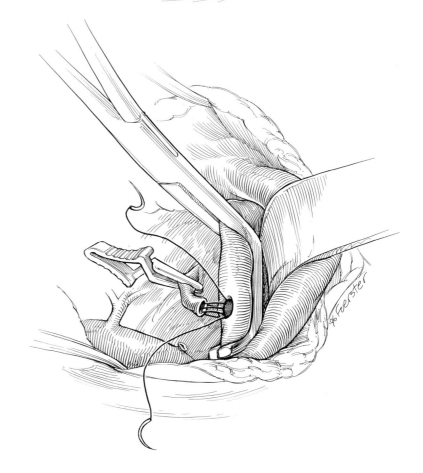

### Figure 212

An end-to-side vertebral to carotid anastomosis is constructed with fine polypropylene suture.

## *Vertebral to Carotid Transposition*

After carefully assessing the best location to avoid kinking of the vertebral artery, a small ellipse of arterial wall is excised from the common carotid artery, and an end-to-side anastomosis is constructed with 6-0 or 7-0 polypropylene suture. The parachuting technique may be useful for at least the posterior hemicircumference of the anastomosis. On completion of the anastomosis (Fig. 213), care must be taken to prevent air and debris from entering the vertebral or distal carotid circulation.

The wound is closed using running suture for the platysma and cutaneous layers. Postoperative wound drainage is routinely employed and is removed after the absence of significant lymphatic leakage has been confirmed.

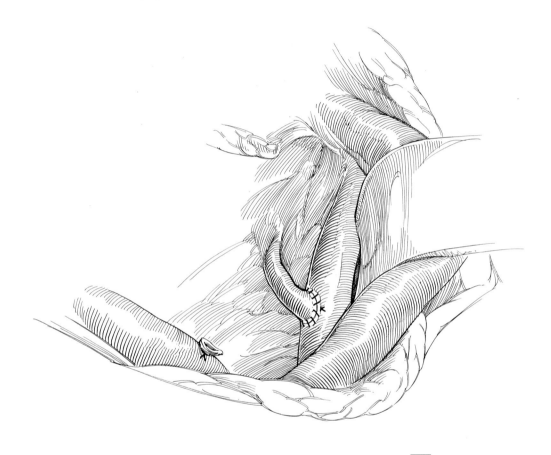

## Figure 213

The completed anastomosis, without twists or kinks in the vertebral artery.

# CHAPTER 32

# Axilloaxillary Bypass

Patients with proximal subclavian occlusive disease may present with symptoms of arm claudication, digital ischemia caused by embolic events, posterior cerebral embolic stroke, or vertebrobasilar symptoms from posterior cerebral hypoperfusion. Bypass from the ascending aorta is the primary choice for treating patients with symptomatic multivessel brachiocephalic or innominate arterial occlusive disease.

Axilloaxillary bypass is an alternative for patients who would poorly tolerate median sternotomy. Its main advantages are superficial dissection, possibility of performing the procedure under local anesthesia, and usefulness in patients who have had previous neck operations or irradiation. The procedure is inappropriate for patients experiencing embolic events from the proximal subclavian or innominate artery, because without ligation, embolic foci are not excluded from the path of blood flow.

## OPERATIVE PROCEDURE

The axillary arteries are exposed through bilateral infraclavicular incisions (Fig. 214). The pectoralis major fascia is divided, and the fibers of the muscle are separated. Immediately beneath the pectoralis major muscle lies the clavipectoral fascia. After it is incised, the surgeon can encircle the pectoralis minor muscle with the index finger (Fig. 215). Division of the pectoralis minor muscle is the key to exposure of the axillary artery. Using electrocautery, the muscle is divided near its insertion on the coracoid process, where the triangularly shaped muscle is relatively narrow; division exposes the axillary artery immediately below. Although the axillary artery lies just posterior and cephalad to the large axillary vein, the vein itself is not always visualized.

Branches of this segment of the axillary artery, such as the thoracoacromial and subscapular arteries, must be controlled to isolate an adequate length for anastomosis. After this is done, the axillary artery segment is controlled with vessel loops or vascular clamps.

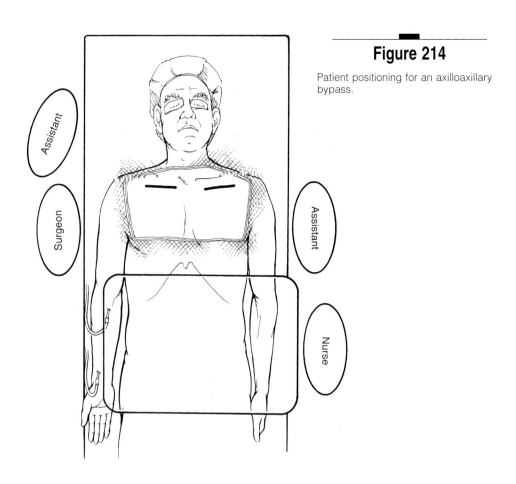

## Figure 214

Patient positioning for an axilloaxillary bypass.

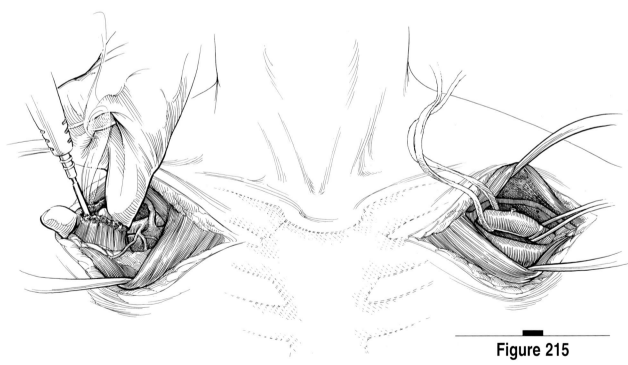

## Figure 215

The axillary arteries are exposed through infraclavicular incisions, cutting the pectoralis minor muscle to expose the midportion of each vessel. Small branches are ligated and divided; larger branches are controlled with vessel loops or fine bulldog clamps.

The use of a vascular clamp with a Satinsky configuration may allow simultaneous control of the axillary artery and its branches without individually clamping each branch (Fig. 216). An 8-mm ePTFE or polyester graft is appropriate as a conduit. After adequate heparinization is achieved, an arteriotomy is made on the anterosuperior surface of the axillary artery, being careful not to incise the posterior wall, which may tent up from the tortuosity created by mobilization and clamping. The anastomosis is completed with 5-0 or 6-0 polypropylene suture, beginning at the midportion of the arteriotomy, continuing around the toe and heel, and tying the suture at the opposite midpoint. The anastomosis is configured in a manner that allows the graft to rise out of the depths of the wound in a gentle arc and without kinking.

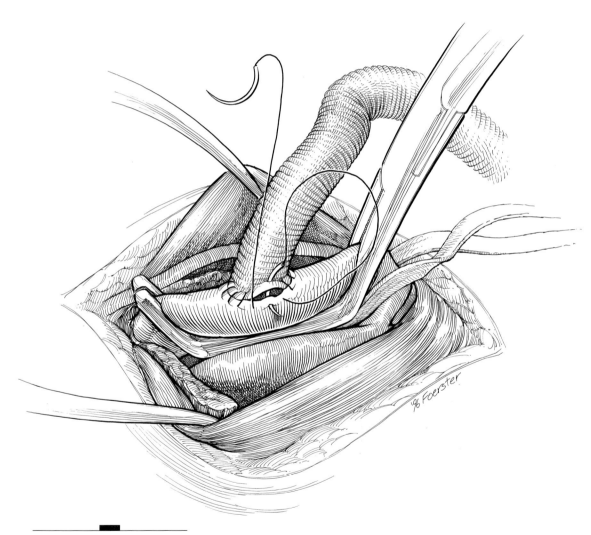

## Figure 216

The proximal anastomosis is sewn in an end-to-side fashion.

## *Axilloaxillary Bypass*

The graft is tunneled subcutaneously across the manubrium (Fig. 217). The distal anastomosis is constructed in an end-to-side fashion in a manner similar to that employed for the proximal anastomosis, except that it is more acutely angled toward the outflow vessel (Fig. 218). Before releasing the proximal clamp and tying down the final sutures, all air and debris must be flushed out of the conduit to prevent emboli from reaching the posterior cerebral circulation through the vertebral artery on the side of the occlusion (Fig. 219).

The pulse at the wrist is palpated at the conclusion of the procedure. The wounds are closed with an absorbable suture for the pectoralis major fascia, followed by closure of the skin. It is not unusual for a small pressure gradient to persist after an axilloaxillary bypass. The large outflow bed of the forequarter, chest, and vertebrobasilar system may be associated with flow rates sufficient to produce a pressure drop if a small-diameter conduit has been used, if the graft is kinked near the proximal anastomosis, or if unsuspected narrowing of the donor vessel exists. This may in part explain the poorer patency rate of axilloaxillary bypass compared with inflow from the ascending aorta. When detected, a significant pressure gradient may be a harbinger of early graft failure and should be addressed.

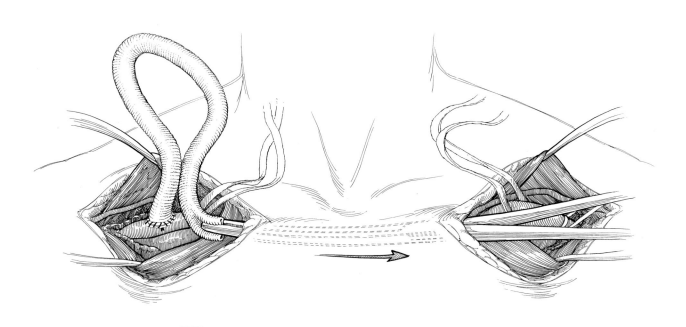

## Figure 217

The graft is tunneled subcutaneously across the manubrium sternum to reach the outflow vessel.

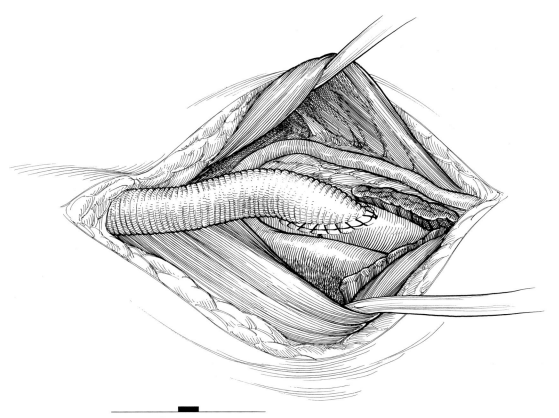

**Figure 218**

The distal anastomosis is completed in
an end-to-side manner.

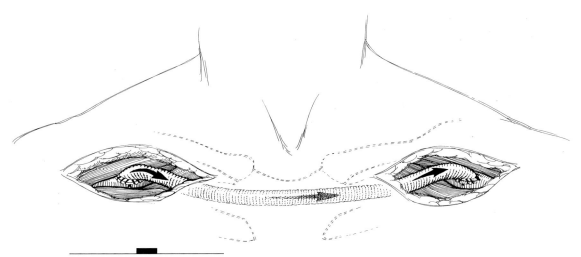

**Figure 219**

On completion of the anastomoses, the
clamps are released, removing the
recipient side proximal axillary artery
clamp last to prevent embolization of air
or debris to the vertebral circulation.

# CHAPTER 33

# Subclavian to Subclavian Bypass

Extrathoracic carotid to subclavian bypass has become the standard procedure for treating symptomatic disease of an isolated proximal subclavian artery. Proximal carotid disease, however, precludes the use of the common carotid artery for inflow. Patients with multivessel brachiocephalic arterial occlusive disease are best treated with an in-line anatomic construction from the ascending aorta. Patients with contraindications to median sternotomy are exceptions to this recommendation, and an axilloaxillary or subclavian to subclavian bypass may be employed in patients with severe pulmonary disease or those who have had previous cardiac surgery. A subclavian to subclavian bypass is shorter and more direct, and it does not interfere with performance of a future median sternotomy. The possibility of bilateral phrenic neuropraxia with the subclavian procedure must be weighed against a somewhat lower patency rate with the axillary approach. The subclavian to subclavian bypass may be advantageous in selected subgroups, such as patients who have had infraclavicular vascular procedures.

## ■ OPERATIVE PROCEDURE

The procedure is performed with the patient in a supine position and after sterile prepping and draping of the neck and upper chest. Bilateral transverse supraclavicular incisions are made (Fig. 220). The subclavian arteries are approached by dividing the lateral head of the sternocleidomastoid muscle, the omohyoid muscle, and the scalene fat pad. The phrenic nerve is identified as it courses along the anterior surface of the anterior scalene muscle. The muscle is divided, being extremely careful to protect the nerve from injury. Immediately beneath the anterior scalene muscle is the subclavian artery, lying somewhat higher in the neck on the right side than the left. The subclavian artery is dissected free of surrounding tissue for a distance of several centimeters. Cephalad branches of the subclavian artery are ligated with silk suture and divided. Frequently, the thyrocervical trunk is sacrificed, as may be the costocervical trunk.

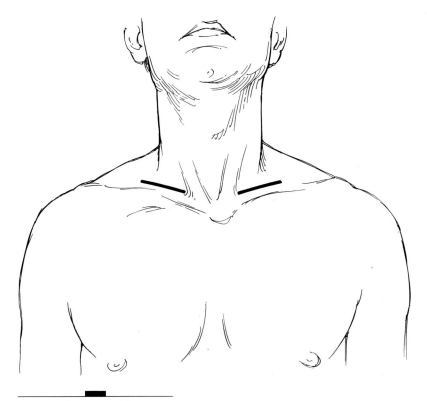

## Figure 220

The incisions used for a subclavian to subclavian bypass are placed in the supraclavicular fossae, approximately 1 cm above the level of the clavicle.

## Subclavian to Subclavian Bypass

The patient is administered heparin, and the subclavian vessels are clamped or occluded with vessel loops (Fig. 221). An incision is made along the anterior aspect of the subclavian artery, and an anastomosis is constructed with 5-0 or 6-0 polypropylene suture. Typically, a 6- or 8-mm, externally supported ePTFE graft is employed, but a polyester conduit may be used with similar results.

The graft is occluded with a Fogarty clamp after completion of the proximal anastomosis. The graft is then tunneled subcutaneously (Fig. 222), and the distal anastomosis is constructed in an end-to-side fashion (Fig. 223). The clamps are released, taking care to release the proximal clamp on the recipient subclavian vessel last to prevent air and debris from entering the posterior cerebral circulation.

Postoperative wound drainage is employed. The wounds are closed in two layers: platysma and skin. The patency of the reconstruction is documented by comparing the right and left brachial blood pressures. The supraclavicular drains are removed as soon as drainage has decreased to less than 15 ml per 8-hour shift.

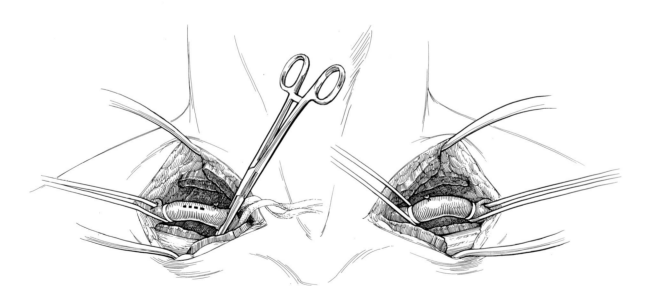

### Figure 221

The right subclavian artery has been exposed and is controlled with a vascular clamp proximally and a Potts tied vessel loop distally. The left subclavian artery is controlled with two Potts tied vessel loops.

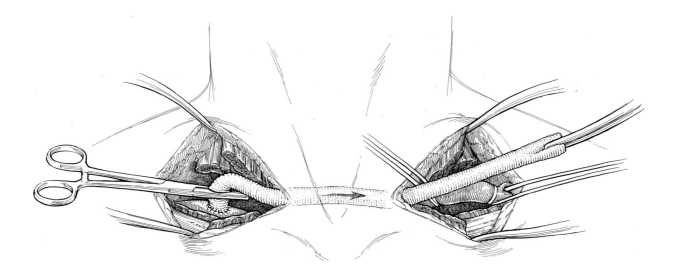

## Figure 222

After the anastomosis to the donor vessel is completed, the graft is clamped proximally and tunneled subcutaneously across the trachea to the recipient subclavian vessel.

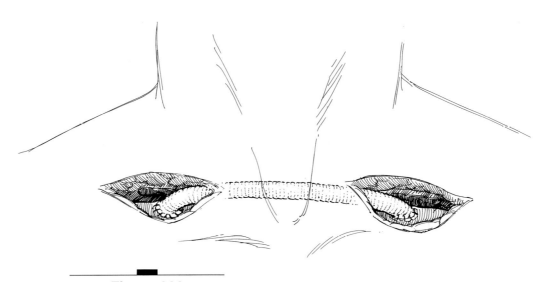

## Figure 223

The completed bypass procedure, with the graft running subcutaneously over the trachea.

# CHAPTER 34

# Ascending Aorta to Carotid Bypass

The low morbidity and excellent long-term results of the extrathoracic carotid to subclavian reconstruction has greatly lessened the need for intrathoracic exposures when treating brachiocephalic arterial disease. Nevertheless, concurrent proximal common carotid and subclavian occlusive disease necessitates the use of an alternative inflow site. The "dome" of the aortic arch is usually involved in patients with this pattern of atherosclerosis, but the proximal ascending aorta is usually relatively spared and therefore represents an ideal choice. Multiple bypasses to the subclavian arteries from the ascending aorta are commonly used to treat nonspecific aortoarteritis or Takayasu's disease.

The technique of exposure and side clamping the ascending aorta reflect experience gained from aortocoronary artery bypass. The median sternotomy is well tolerated by most patients and is associated with a low incidence of postoperative pain and wound complications. In contrast, the use of the descending aorta as an inflow site for brachiocephalic reconstruction requires a left thoracotomy, a more painful incision that is less well tolerated by patients with pulmonary disease. Moreover, the decubitus position seriously limits exposure of the cervical portions of the carotid and subclavian arteries.

The specific bypass configuration is dictated by the location of the occlusive disease, but several caveats are warranted. First, the size of the thoracic outlet must be considered when planning the bypass. For instance, few patients can tolerate more than two grafts passing up into the neck without developing postoperative airway or swallowing difficulties. Even two grafts may cause difficulties in some. Reconstruction of multiple vessels may therefore require a combination of intrathoracic and extrathoracic bypass limbs. Second, cerebral ischemia with proximal brachiocephalic clamping is rare, and monitoring in the form of intraoperative electroencephalography or routine shunting is unnecessary. Third, long prosthetic graft limbs to the carotid bifurcation may be associated with a higher than expected incidence of perioperative and postoperative neurologic events, presumably from the formation and subsequent embolization of platelet thrombi from the lining of the prosthesis. This observation has led some surgeons to perform a shorter bypass to the proximal common carotid artery with a separate carotid bifurcation endarterectomy when treating patients with tandem lesions. Fourth, the postoperative hyperperfusion syndrome characterized by headache, seizures, and intracranial hemorrhage is especially common among patients with multiple, high-grade brachiocephalic stenoses.

## OPERATIVE PROCEDURE

The patient is in the supine position, with the neck hyperextended. The endotracheal tube is secured in a sagittal plane over the nose to allow it to be draped out of the sterile field. The operation is begun with a standard median sternotomy, and in the example featured, bilateral cervical incisions are made along the anterior border of the sternocleidomastoid muscles (Fig. 224). The superior mediastinal fat and thymus are divided, taking care to avoid injury to the crossing left brachiocephalic vein. The pericardial sac is identified and incised in its superior portion, exposing the bulging ascending aorta. The vessel is carefully cleared of areolar attachments, exposing the anterior two thirds of its circumference for a length of several centimeters.

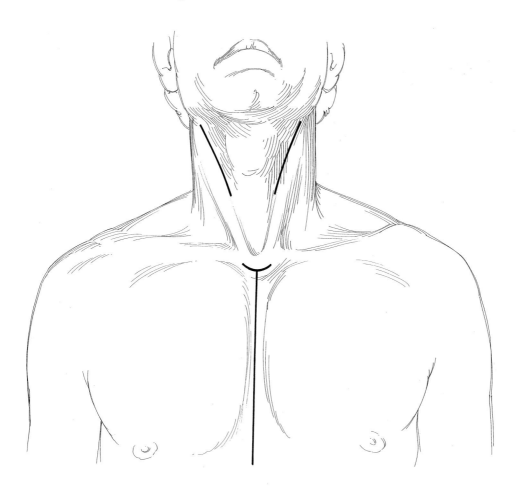

**Figure 224**

The patient is positioned supine, with hyperextension of the neck in preparation for aortocarotid bypass. The three incision sites are indicated.

## Ascending Aorta to Carotid Bypass

The carotid bifurcations are exposed in the usual fashion, although the inability to turn the head to the side keeps the bifurcation in a direct anteroposterior plane, with the external carotid and superior thyroid arteries obscuring the exposure of the internal carotid artery. More extensive dissection and mobilization of the bifurcation vessels is often required to improve visualization of the internal carotid artery.

The patient is administered heparin and short-acting vasodilators as needed to lower the systemic pressure and allow safe aortic clamping. The ascending aorta is partially occluded with a side-biting clamp while observing changes in systemic arterial pressure and assessing the degree of ventricular dilatation with transesophageal echocardiography, if available. Temporary internal carotid clamping during the application of the aortic clamp may lessen the risk of cerebral embolization from unexpected aortic atheromatous debris.

A bifurcated graft is chosen, keeping the diameter of the graft's body at 12 or 14 mm to limit the size of the aortotomy. This provides a better match with the outflow vessels and lessens the bulk of the prosthetic limbs exiting the thoracic outlet. The graft is beveled to 45° and tunneled beneath the left brachiocephalic vein to the cervical wounds. The proximal anastomosis is completed with 3-0 or 4-0 suture, and the aortic clamp is carefully released (Fig. 225). Pledgeted repair sutures are placed as necessary.

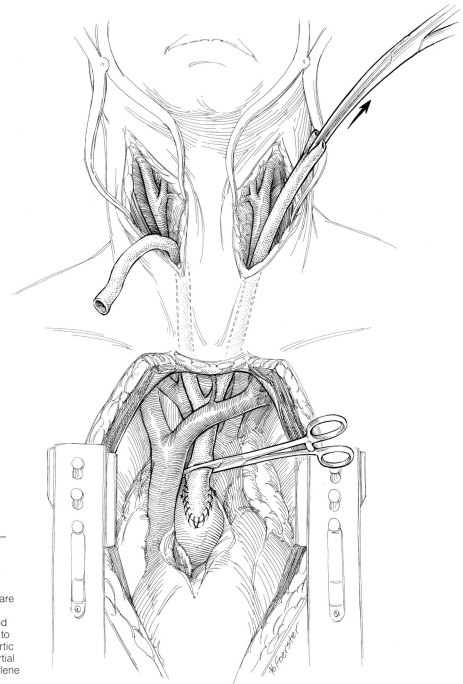

**Figure 225**

The ascending aorta is exposed after incising the superior portion of the pericardium. The carotid bifurcations are exposed through separate cervical incisions. A bifurcated graft is tunneled beneath the left brachiocephalic vein to reach the carotid bifurcations. The aortic anastomosis is constructed with a partial occlusion clamp, using 3-0 polypropylene suture.

## *Ascending Aorta to Carotid Bypass*

Carotid endarterectomies are individually performed when necessary, anastomosing the limbs of the graft over each endarterectomy site with 5-0 or 6-0 polypropylene suture. The hoods of the anastomoses are fashioned to function as patches for the endarterectomies (Fig. 226). An end-to-end anastomosis is appropriate in the presence of embolizing proximal carotid stenotic lesions, but an end-to-side configuration is performed in the absence of prior emboli or when the common carotid artery is chronically occluded.

Various patterns of occlusive lesions may be encountered. For multiple proximal occlusions of brachiocephalic arteries, as is often the case in Takayasu's aortoarteritis, other combinations of aorta-based bypasses can be used (Fig. 227). Bypass is confined to the vessels for which a substantive clinical gain from revascularization can be predicted.

Flow is restored to the carotid circulation after flushing air and debris out of the graft limbs, remembering that ePTFE and coated polyester grafts may be impervious to air and that puncture with a needle at the highest portion of the graft may be necessary for complete evacuation. A single mediastinal drainage tube is placed.

The wounds are closed after ensuring the absence of technical defects with intraoperative Doppler ultrasonography, duplex scanning, or arteriographic interrogation. Patients with multiple critical occlusive lesions are closely followed postoperatively. Fluids are restricted in those with persistently high duplex velocities, and mannitol is administered if signs and symptoms of cerebral hyperperfusion develop.

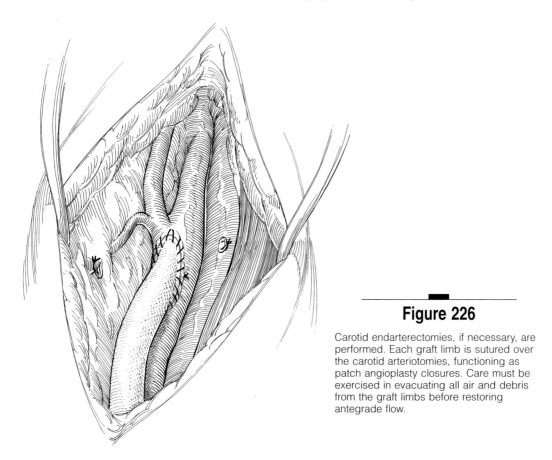

### Figure 226

Carotid endarterectomies, if necessary, are performed. Each graft limb is sutured over the carotid arteriotomies, functioning as patch angioplasty closures. Care must be exercised in evacuating all air and debris from the graft limbs before restoring antegrade flow.

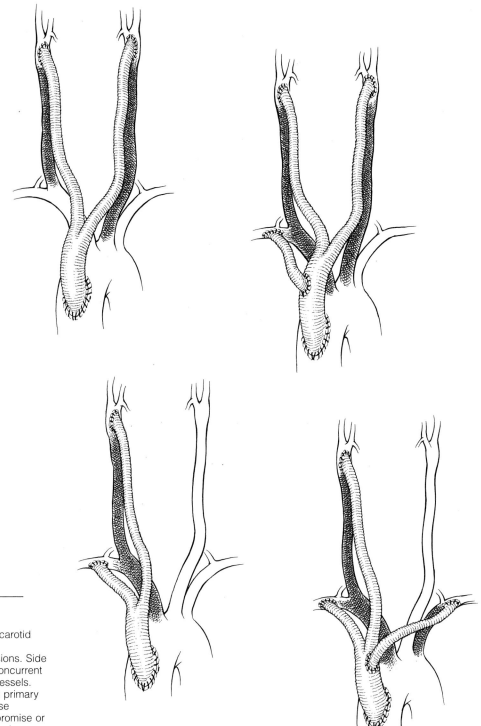

## Figure 227

A variety of options exist for aortocarotid
reconstruction, depending on the
configuration of the arterial occlusions. Side
limbs may be added to provide concurrent
reconstruction of the subclavian vessels.
The size of the thoracic outlet is a primary
consideration in the design of these
procedures, and respiratory compromise or
swallowing difficulties may develop in some
cases.

# CHAPTER 35

# *Innominate Endarterectomy*

Innominate endarterectomy may be employed to address localized innominate atheromatous disease (Fig. 228). The procedure is unsafe when the disease extends to the aortic arch, because application of a proximal side-biting aortic clamp causes fracture of the aortic wall and risks uncontrollable hemorrhage, distal embolization, or dissection (Fig. 229). The infrequent use of innominate endarterectomy is a direct result of the rarity of localized disease, and most patients require a bypass graft originating on the ascending aorta or one of the contralateral brachiocephalic arteries.

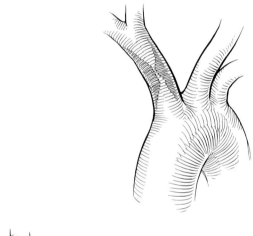

## Figure 228

An innominate endarterectomy may be considered when localized disease does not involve the aortic arch.

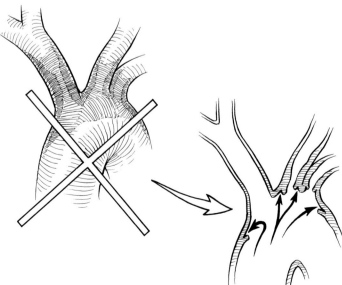

## Figure 229

The procedure is unsafe when the atherosclerotic disease is diffuse. Plaque fracture may result in dissection, distal embolization, or hemorrhage.

## OPERATIVE PROCEDURE

In appropriate candidates, an innominate endarterectomy can be a rewarding undertaking, eliminating an embolic source without the use of a bypass conduit. A median sternotomy provides the best exposure, but more limited incisions such as an upper sternotomy or clavicular resection have been used. The pericardium is incised, the left brachiocephalic vein is mobilized and retracted out of the way, and the proximal right subclavian and common carotid arteries are controlled. Care is taken to protect the recurrent laryngeal nerve as it courses around the proximal subclavian artery. A partially occluding aortic clamp is placed after adequate heparinization and distal clamping (Fig. 230).

An endarterectomy is performed, taking care to protect the fragile innominate artery wall from inadvertent injury. In most cases, the innominate artery is large enough to close primarily, but small vessels may be closed with a prosthetic patch.

Air and debris are evacuated before restoring distal flow. The surgeon must protect the subclavian artery from embolization, just as the carotid artery is protected, because vertebral emboli and posterior cerebral infarction may have devastating consequences. Heparin is reversed with protamine sulfate titrated to the activated clotting time. The sternotomy is closed over a single mediastinal tube.

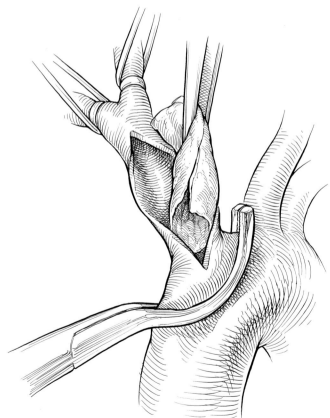

### Figure 230

After distal vascular control, a side-biting aortic clamp is applied. A longitudinal innominate arteriotomy is made, and an endarterectomy is performed. The artery is usually large enough to allow safe primary closure; alternatively, a prosthetic patch can be employed.

# CHAPTER 36

# Ascending Aorta to Innominate Bypass

Patients with disease of the proximal innominate artery are candidates for the construction of a bypass between the ascending aorta and the innominate bifurcation. This procedure is easier and safer than an innominate endarterectomy, because it avoids clamping of the aorta at the level of the innominate artery takeoff.

## OPERATIVE PROCEDURE

The patient is positioned with the neck turned to the left, in case exposure of the right carotid or subclavian artery becomes necessary (Fig. 231). Through a median sternotomy, the mediastinal fat and thymic remnant are dissected off the vascular structures. The left brachiocephalic vein is cleared of surrounding tissue, ligating small branches as necessary to obtain additional exposure (Fig. 232). Cephalad retraction of the brachiocephalic vein and incision of the superior-most portion of the pericardial sac provides excellent exposure of a length of ascending aorta suitable for the anastomosis. The right common carotid and subclavian vessels are controlled (Fig. 233), avoiding injury to the recurrent laryngeal nerve as it hooks beneath the proximal subclavian artery. The patient is administered heparin, and the systemic blood pressure is lowered to facilitate aortic clamping.

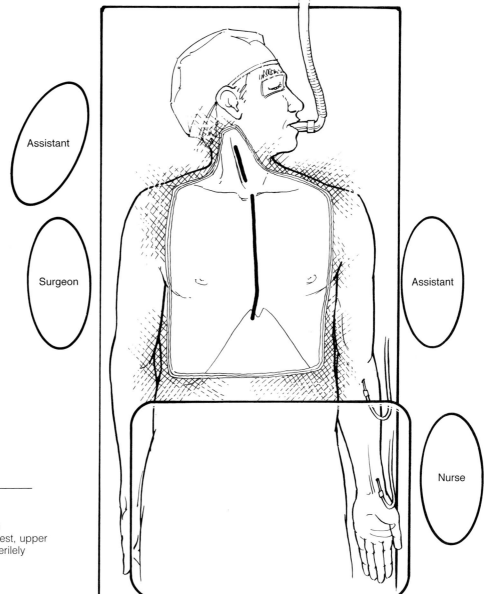

**Figure 231**

In preparation for an innominate endarterectomy, the patient's chest, upper abdomen, and right neck are sterilely prepared and draped.

## Ascending Aorta to Innominate Bypass

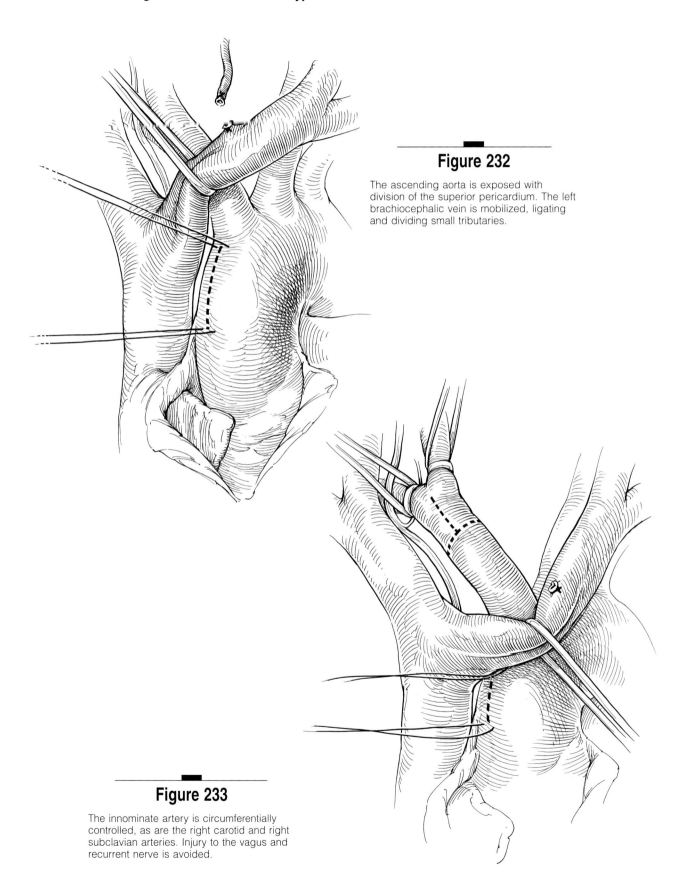

### Figure 232

The ascending aorta is exposed with division of the superior pericardium. The left brachiocephalic vein is mobilized, ligating and dividing small tributaries.

### Figure 233

The innominate artery is circumferentially controlled, as are the right carotid and right subclavian arteries. Injury to the vagus and recurrent nerve is avoided.

A polyester or ePTFE graft is chosen, with a diameter approximating that of the distal innominate artery. The carotid and subclavian vessels are occluded, and a side-biting aortic clamp is applied. An aortotomy is made (Fig. 234), and the proximal anastomosis is constructed with 3-0 or 4-0 suture. The graft is clamped proximally and threaded beneath the left brachiocephalic vein (Fig. 235). The distal innominate artery is transected, the proximal stump is oversewn, and the distal end is beveled (Fig. 236). The distal anastomosis is completed with 4-0 or 5-0 suture, and the air and debris is flushed out of the graft before restoration of blood flow (Fig. 237).

After release of the clamps, adequate antegrade flow is ascertained by palpation of the distal vessels or with intraoperative duplex ultrasonography. Heparin is reversed with protamine sulfate, and the sternotomy is closed over a mediastinal tube. The tube is removed early to lessen the risk of secondarily infecting the graft, and the patient is monitored for signs of cerebral hyperperfusion during the postoperative period.

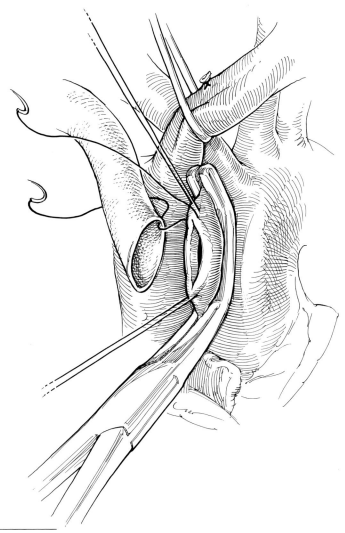

**Figure 234**

An aortic side-biting clamp is applied, and the proximal anastomosis is performed with 4-0 polypropylene suture.

## Ascending Aorta to Innominate Bypass

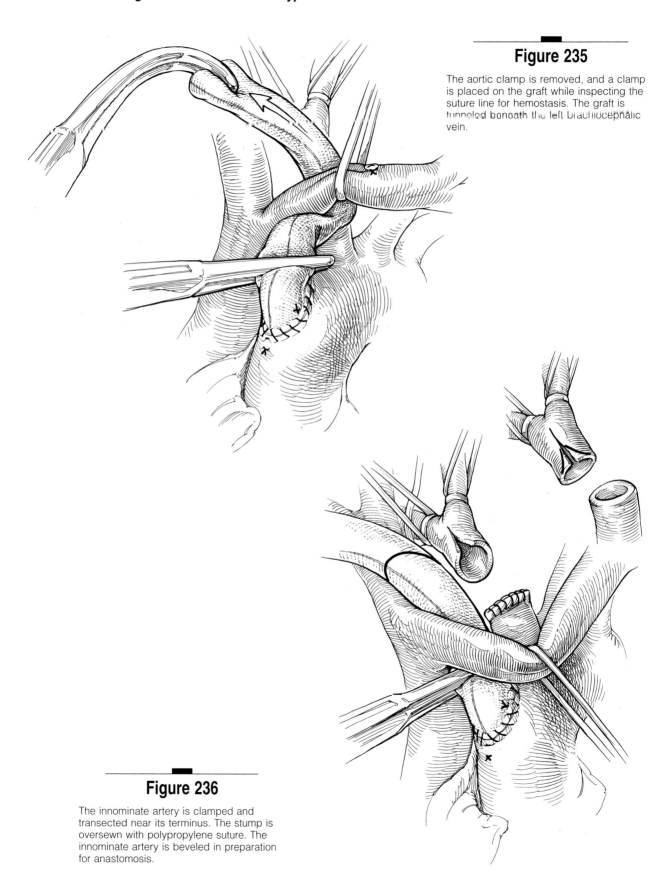

### Figure 235

The aortic clamp is removed, and a clamp is placed on the graft while inspecting the suture line for hemostasis. The graft is tunneled beneath the left brachiocephalic vein.

### Figure 236

The innominate artery is clamped and transected near its terminus. The stump is oversewn with polypropylene suture. The innominate artery is beveled in preparation for anastomosis.

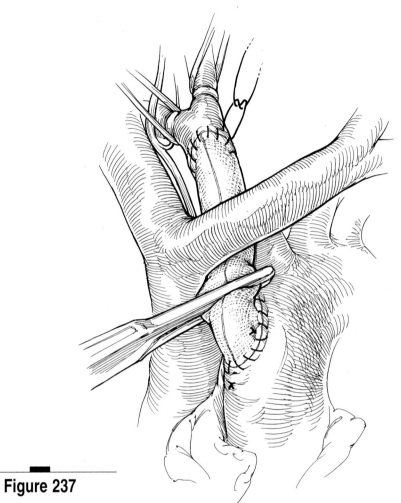

**Figure 237**

The distal anastomosis is completed with 4-0 or 5-0 polypropylene suture. Air and debris are flushed out of the graft before restoring blood flow.

# THORACIC OUTLET SYNDROME

# CHAPTER 37

# Transaxillary First Rib Resection With Sympathectomy

The thoracic outlet syndrome manifests with neurologic, venous, or arterial symptoms caused by compression of various structures as they pass through the thoracic outlet. Compression of the brachial plexus is the most common type of thoracic outlet syndrome, but it is associated with the lowest rate of success after first rib resection. For this reason, patients should be given a thorough trial of exercises directed at improving posture and strengthening the shoulder girdle muscles before considering surgery. Patients with the classic lower cord distribution of symptoms obtain the best results.

Vascular symptoms are infrequently observed in patients with the thoracic outlet syndrome. In contrast to the results obtained for neurologic symptoms, first rib resection is usually successful in relieving venous and arterial symptoms. Arterial symptoms are related to focal compression with poststenotic dilatation, ultimately leading to thromboembolism. They should prompt a search for a cervical rib or an equivalent skeletal abnormality, which almost invariably accompanies *symptomatic* arterial thoracic outlet compression.

There exist a variety of operative options for patients with thoracic outlet syndrome, each of which is directed at decompressing the structures that form the musculoskeletal boundary of the thoracic outlet. Historically, clavicular resection was the most commonly performed procedure, and it still may be appropriate for patients with venous symptoms requiring simultaneous decompression and venous reconstruction. Resection of an anomalous cervical rib is indicated, and it can be accomplished through a transaxillary or supraclavicular approach. Anterior scalenectomy has been advocated for patients with "upper plexus involvement," consisting of pain in the distribution of the C5, C6, and C7 nerve roots.

We avoid the use of anterior scalenectomy for thoracic outlet syndrome, because patients appear to achieve better and longer lasting relief with first rib resection. It provides more reliable thoracic outlet decompression by removing the rib and any related structures (e.g., anterior scalene muscle, anomalous congenital bands, cervical rib remnants) that may contribute to neurovascular impingement.

# OPERATIVE PROCEDURE

## Transaxillary First Rib Resection

A transaxillary route is most efficient for first rib resection. Under general endotracheal anesthesia, the patient is placed in a full lateral decubitus position with the patient's back near the edge of the table (Fig. 238). The head is supported on a pillow to avoid stretching the brachial plexus as the second assistant elevates the arm. The shoulder, back, axilla, and upper arm are sterilely prepared, and the forearm and hand are covered with an impervious stocking. The surgeon stands behind the patient, while the first assistant stands in the front to manipulate the retractors. The second assistant stands next to the surgeon, cradling the patient's arm in his own.

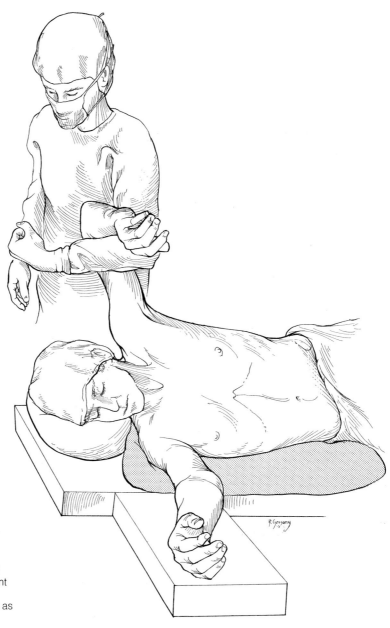

**Figure 238**

The patient is positioned in a full lateral decubitus position. The second assistant cradles the patient's arm to elevate the neurovascular structures off the first rib as appropriate.

## Transaxillary First Rib Resection With Sympathectomy

A transverse incision is made between the latissimus dorsi and pectoralis major muscles, just below the axillary hairline (Fig. 239). Dissection is carried down to the chest wall and serratus anterior muscle. The surgeon gently develops a tunnel to the axilla, pushing the areolar tissue aside. Visualization is improved through the use of a Deaver retractor placed beneath the pectoralis major muscle as the first assistant retracts the muscle medially and anteriorly (Fig. 240). A fiberoptic light may improve visual exposure, although the surgeon can usually achieve adequate visualization through careful placement of high-quality, ceiling-mounted lighting.

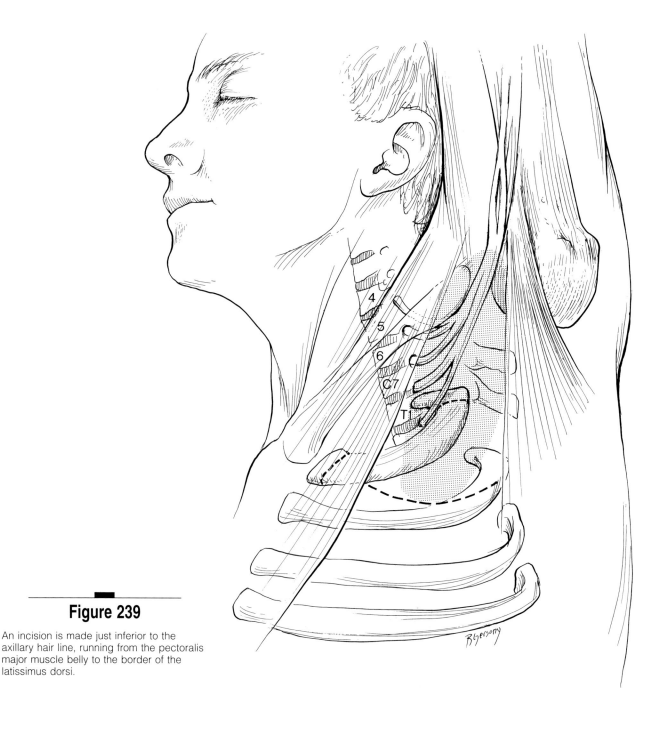

## Figure 239

An incision is made just inferior to the axillary hair line, running from the pectoralis major muscle belly to the border of the latissimus dorsi.

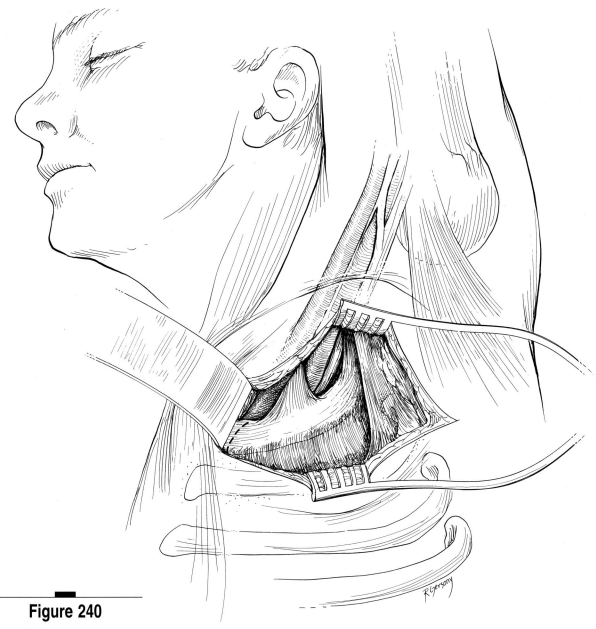

**Figure 240**

After blunt creation of a tunnel to reach the axilla, the first rib is cleared of surrounding fibroadipose tissue. The anterior scalene muscle and its surrounding neurovascular structures are identified.

### *Transaxillary First Rib Resection With Sympathectomy*

An inferior branch of the axillary artery, the supreme thoracic artery, is clipped and divided to allow the surgeon to gently elevate the subclavian artery off the first rib. The subclavian artery and brachial plexus are gently pushed off of the rib with arm retraction and blunt dissection, exposing the upper margin of the rib. The neurovascular structures fall posteriorly off the first rib as the second assistant elevates the patient's arm and shoulder. This maneuver must only be used intermittently to avoid significant postoperative pain and temporary neuropraxic symptoms. The first rib is palpated and cleared of adherent tissue with a periosteal elevator. The middle and posterior scalene muscles are removed from the lateral aspect of the rib with the elevator.

The anterior scalene muscle is visualized as it inserts on the medial aspect of the first rib. A right angle clamp is inserted behind the muscle, and the muscle is divided with the scissors (Fig. 241). The attachments of the intercostal muscle are then lysed from the inferior margin of the rib (Fig. 242), gently developing a plane beneath the rib to depress the pleura from its undersurface. The rib should be completely cleared of soft tissue at this point to allow placement of large rib shears around its anterior-most aspect.

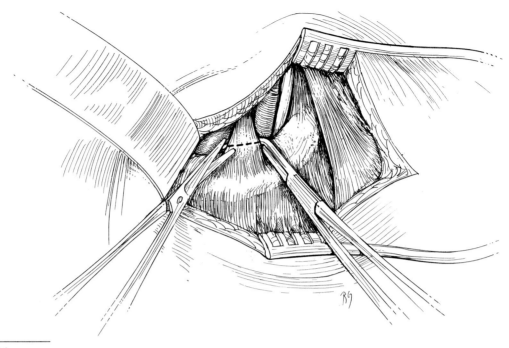

**Figure 241**

The anterior scalene muscle is divided as it
inserts on the first rib.

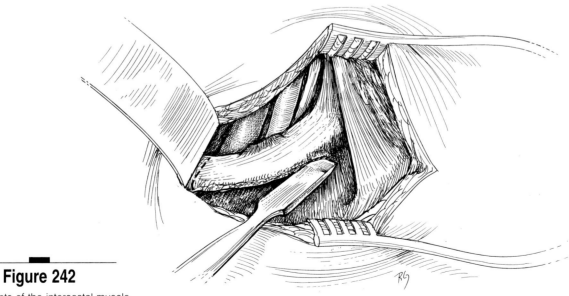

**Figure 242**

The attachments of the intercostal muscle
are cleared from the first rib with a
periosteal elevator. The rib is surrounded
circumferentially, taking care to avoid
inadvertent entry into the pleural space.

## *Transaxillary First Rib Resection With Sympathectomy*

The second assistant elevates the shoulder to retract the subclavian vein away from the rib as the rib is divided. The rib shears is moved to the posterior-most aspect of the rib (Fig. 243). The rib is excised, but additional bone is removed with rongeurs while the brachial plexus is gently retracted and protected with the aid of a spatula (Fig. 244). The bone is excised posteriorly to a level beyond the plexus, keeping the stump of the rib short and smooth to avoid postoperative irritation of the T1 nerve root. Excision of additional rib must be done under direct vision, with constant effort to protect the brachial plexus.

The wound is filled with saline and inspected for persistent bubbling as the anesthesiologist hyperinflates the lung. If a pneumothorax has occurred, the wound is closed over a small catheter, removing the catheter in the recovery room after the incision has been rendered air tight. The subcutaneous tissues are closed with a running absorbable suture, closing the skin with an absorbable subcuticular stitch. A postoperative chest radiograph is obtained in the postanesthesia care unit.

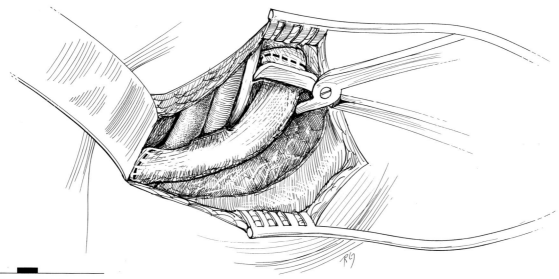

## Figure 243

The second assistant raises the arm, elevating the neurovascular structures off the first rib. The rib is divided anteriorly and posteriorly under direct vision.

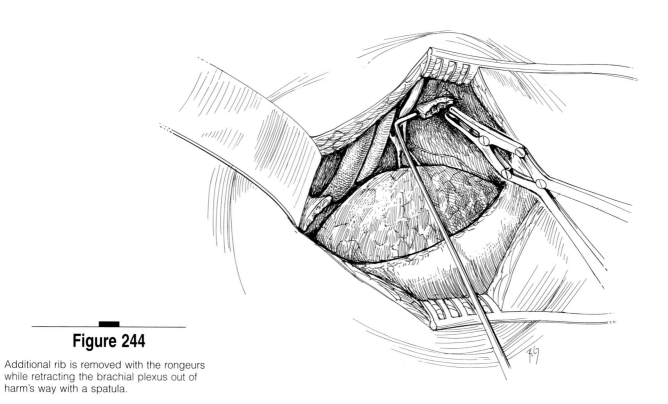

## Figure 244

Additional rib is removed with the rongeurs while retracting the brachial plexus out of harm's way with a spatula.

## Transaxillary Sympathectomy

Some patients with the thoracic outlet syndrome have concurrent vasospastic symptoms; others develop causalgic pain, and those with arterial thromboembolism may suffer small vessel occlusions distally. Any of these clinical presentations may warrant sympathectomy. The transaxillary approach with first rib removal provides a safe and adequate exposure of the stellate and upper thoracic sympathetic ganglia.

After removal of the first rib, the lung is manually depressed away from the posteromedial chest wall (Fig. 245). The stellate ganglion is visualized on the posterior remnant of the first rib. The sympathetic chain runs inferiorly and laterally, coursing over the posterior neck of each rib. The caudal one third (i.e., T1 portion) of the stellate ganglion is excised, along with the T2 and T3 ganglia. Careful examination reveals mild, usually temporary Horner's syndrome symptoms in many patients. Although a relatively low incidence of permanent Horner's syndrome has been reported in the literature, the patient should be warned of this possibility.

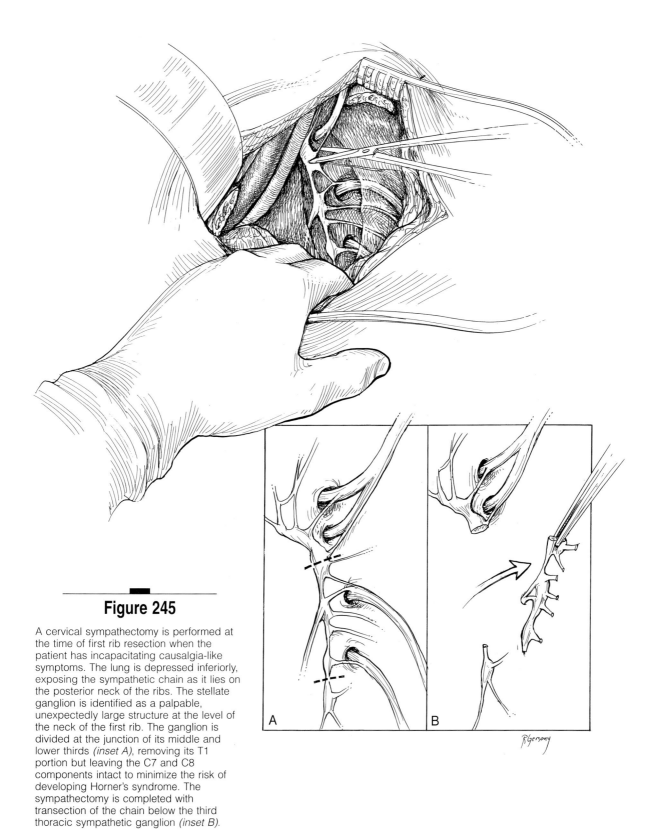

**Figure 245**

A cervical sympathectomy is performed at the time of first rib resection when the patient has incapacitating causalgia-like symptoms. The lung is depressed inferiorly, exposing the sympathetic chain as it lies on the posterior neck of the ribs. The stellate ganglion is identified as a palpable, unexpectedly large structure at the level of the neck of the first rib. The ganglion is divided at the junction of its middle and lower thirds *(inset A)*, removing its T1 portion but leaving the C7 and C8 components intact to minimize the risk of developing Horner's syndrome. The sympathectomy is completed with transection of the chain below the third thoracic sympathetic ganglion *(inset B)*.

# VENOUS PROCEDURES

# CHAPTER 38

# Varicose Vein Excision

Varicose veins of the leg that develop spontaneously, without previous deep venous thrombosis or other pathologic conditions, are called primary varicosities. The cause of primary varicose veins is unclear but is probably related to congenital incompetence or absence of key venous valves such as those that guard the entry of the superficial into the deep system. Superficial varicosities resulting from increased pressure and reflux after deep venous thrombosis are called secondary varicose veins.

The two general indications for varicose vein surgery are relief of symptoms (e.g., pain, swelling, stasis change or bleeding from an eroding varix) and cosmetic deformity. The best candidates for varicose vein excision are those with a normal deep venous system, without valvular incompetence of the deep or perforating veins. The status of the deep, perforating, and superficial veins is readily established with noninvasive methods such as plethysmography, Doppler examination, and duplex ultrasonography.

Unless the procedure is done for cosmetic indications, varicose vein excision should be undertaken only after an adequate trial of nonoperative therapy. Patients should be given a graded compression stocking with an applied pressure of 30 mm Hg or greater. Elevation of the extremity at intervals during the day and night can lessen edema. The patient should limit activities requiring prolonged standing. Although these measures do not decrease the size or number of the patient's varicose veins, they occasionally provide enough symptomatic relief that an operation is no longer necessary, which may be important when managing older patients.

When intervention for varicose veins is elected, several options may be used singly or in combination. These procedures are intended to correct or improve the abnormal hemodynamics or to remove or obliterate the varicose veins. High ligation of the greater and/or lesser saphenous vein flush with its junction with the femoral or popliteal vein is the mainstay of the corrective approach. This approach is designed to prevent sapheno-femoral or saphenopopliteal reflux, and it is mandatory when such reflux exists. In some cases of *early* varicose veins for which isolated and uncomplicated saphenofemoral reflux is found to be the underlying cause, high ligation alone or combined with local excision or sclerotherapy of visible varicosities may suffice. More often, high ligation and local excision should be combined with stripping of the greater saphenous vein from the ankle or from the knee to the groin. Leaving the upper segment in place may lead to recurrences.

Having addressed the greater saphenous vein, the remaining options concern how to remove or obliterate the visible varicosities. These saphenous venous tributaries are often the patient's major focus and are not removed by greater saphenous stripping alone. Instead, they are controlled by local excision or sclerotherapy. Local excision may be performed cosmetically by using multiple small stab incisions at premarked sites.

Alternatively, sclerotherapy may be used at the time of operation and postoperatively. It is effective, with reasonably little local reaction, only if the "empty vein" technique is used and multiple small aliquots (0.3 to 0.9 ml of sclerosant) are injected, followed by compression. Even then, this approach is suitable mainly for small varicosities. The technique is quite different from that used for telangiectasias or "spider veins," for which 0.1 to 0.2 ml of sclerosant or hypertonic (e.g., 24%) saline are injected with 27- or 30-gauge needles.

# OPERATIVE PROCEDURE

Extensive varicosities involving the greater saphenous system require the classic procedure of high ligation and stripping. The procedure is done under regional or general anesthesia after marking accessory venous branches with an indelible pen. The greater saphenous vein is exposed just anterior to the medial malleolus (Fig. 246). The vein is ligated and divided, and an internal stripper is passed through the vein to its terminus. A short transverse groin incision is made to expose the saphenofemoral junction, and all saphenous venous tributaries are ligated and divided at that location. The saphenofemoral junction is ligated flush with the femoral vein.

The patient is placed in a full Trendelenburg position, and the stripper is pulled from the groin while holding pressure over the medial calf and thigh as a hemostatic maneuver. Accessory varicosities are excised through small incisions after removal of the saphenous vein. These techniques are described separately later. Stripping of the lesser saphenous vein can be accomplished at the same time by passing the stripper from the lateral malleolar area to the saphenopopliteal junction. The incisions are closed, and a compression bandage is applied.

Lesser procedures may be employed for the treatment of superficial varicosities when the greater saphenous vein is normal or at least when saphenofemoral reflux is not the culprit. The advantage of such limited procedures is that they spare the vein for subsequent use as a bypass conduit. These ambulatory surgical procedures remove the accessory varicosities through small incisions and preserve the saphenous vein (Fig. 247).

For excision through small incisions, the varicosities are marked preoperatively with the patient in the standing position. The leg is sterilely prepared after the induction of general or regional anesthesia, although a few limited excisions may be performed with local anesthesia alone. Small incisions are placed over the varicosities. The veins are dissected free of surrounding tissue with the scissors, retracting the skin with a vein retractor or skin hook (see Fig. 247, inset A). Venous tributaries are ligated or clipped. Usually, several centimeters of vein can be removed before another incision is necessary. Each incision is closed with interrupted absorbable sutures, and the legs are covered with compression bandages.

The stab avulsion technique is used as an alternative to excision through small incisions. It is most appropriate when the primary indication for excision is cosmetic but is also appropriate as an adjunct to greater saphenous high ligation and stripping. The patient is placed in a steep Trendelenburg position. Tiny incisions are made over the previously marked varicosities using a No. 11 knife blade (see Fig. 247, inset B). The varix is grasped with a mosquito clamp and gently rocked from side to side, delivering a length of vein into the wound. The varix is tugged and finally avulsed. The assistant holds pressure on the stab wound until bleeding ceases. The process is repeated, spacing stab incisions as necessary to remove the veins.

The incisions are small enough that sutures are unnecessary; each wound is closed with a single Steri-Strip. Compression bandages are applied. The stab avulsion method is associated with minimal postoperative pain and provides an excellent cosmetic result.

## *Varicose Vein Excision*

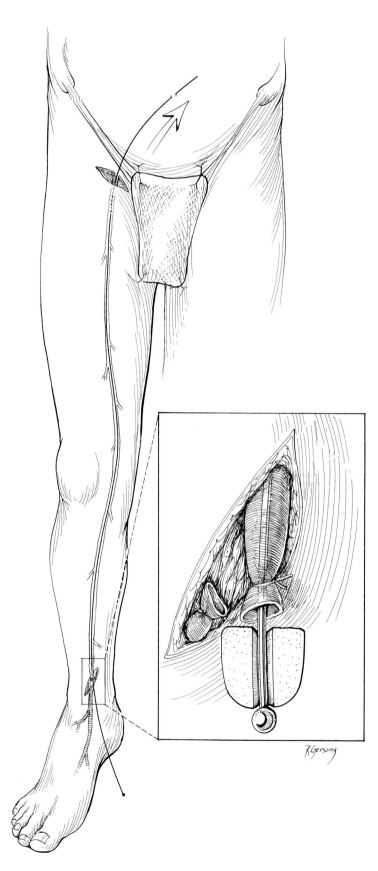

## Figure 246

The traditional method of addressing
varicose veins begins with stripping of the
greater saphenous vein. The vein is
exposed through a small groin incision, and
an incision is placed just anterior to the
medial malleolus. The plastic rod is
threaded from the foot to the groin. The vein
is tied over the rod, and the bullet is
attached *(inset)*. The patient is placed in a
steep Trendelenburg position, and the vein
is stripped as the instrument is withdrawn.

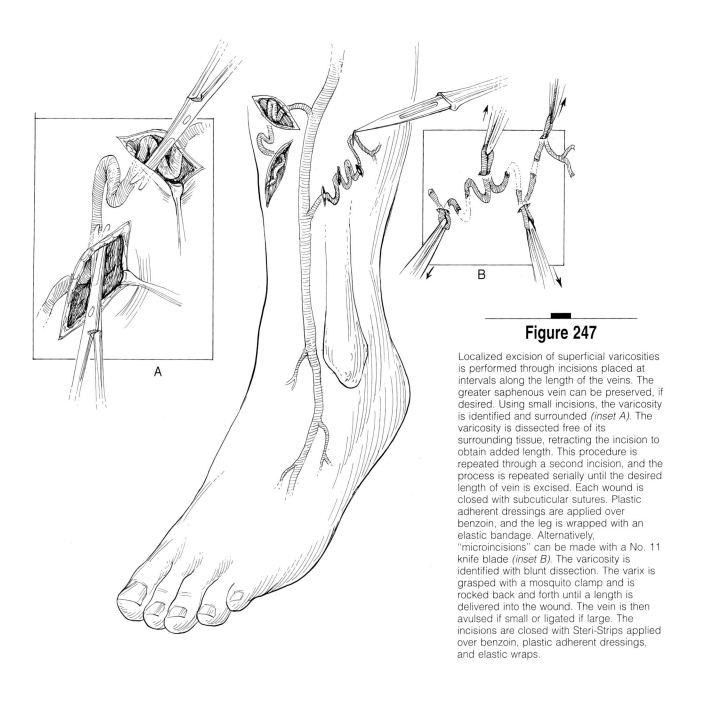

**Figure 247**

Localized excision of superficial varicosities is performed through incisions placed at intervals along the length of the veins. The greater saphenous vein can be preserved, if desired. Using small incisions, the varicosity is identified and surrounded *(inset A)*. The varicosity is dissected free of its surrounding tissue, retracting the incision to obtain added length. This procedure is repeated through a second incision, and the process is repeated serially until the desired length of vein is excised. Each wound is closed with subcuticular sutures. Plastic adherent dressings are applied over benzoin, and the leg is wrapped with an elastic bandage. Alternatively, "microincisions" can be made with a No. 11 knife blade *(inset B)*. The varicosity is identified with blunt dissection. The varix is grasped with a mosquito clamp and is rocked back and forth until a length is delivered into the wound. The vein is then avulsed if small or ligated if large. The incisions are closed with Steri-Strips applied over benzoin, plastic adherent dressings, and elastic wraps.

A

B

# CHAPTER 39

# Venous Valve Transposition

The signs of chronic venous insufficiency consist of brawny edema of the leg, low-grade inflammation, brownish discoloration of the pretibial skin as a result of extravasated red blood cells, and ultimately, ulceration. These sequelae have been called the post-thrombotic syndrome, although as many as two-thirds of the affected individuals have no history of deep venous thrombosis.

Most large practices encounter a variable proportion of patients with primary rather than secondary chronic venous insufficiency. The former fare better after venous reconstructive procedures, partly because of the availability of valvuloplasty as an option. The hemodynamic derangements underlying this complex picture consist of venous valvular incompetence and, in some patients, venous outflow obstruction. Whereas outflow obstruction can be treated by recanalization of the obstructed venous segment or venous bypass (see Chapter 41), valvular incompetence requires the creation of one or more functional valves to combat reflux.

No venous reconstructive procedure should be considered until a thorough trial of conservative measures, such as elevation, local wound care, and compression stockings, has been completely exhausted. Therapeutic intervention in patients with incapacitating symptoms must be preceded by a full diagnostic workup to identify the underlying anatomic abnormalities. Ascending venography, probably the most commonly performed test, is of little value in defining anything other than the extent of venous thrombosis. However, functional studies such as ambulatory venous pressure monitoring and its noninvasive correlates, air and photoplethysmography, provide some quantification of the severity of venous valvular reflux. Duplex ultrasonography, with measurement of valve closing times, has in some centers supplanted the earlier techniques, relying on valve closure time to identify patients with significant incompetence. The test is also useful in assessing the success of venous valve interposition.

When the results of functional studies are clearly abnormal, ascending and descending forms of venography are required before operative intervention. The ascending study defines the patency of the venous system, outlining the extent of any obstruction. Descending venography visualizes retrograde flow through the deep venous system, documenting the presence or absence of valvular incompetence, and demonstrates anatomic abnormalities at each successive level. Incompetent but otherwise preserved valves, as seen in primary valvular incompetence, can be directly addressed with valvuloplasty. Commonly, the entire valve structure has been destroyed during thrombosis and recanalization, and transposition of a functionally intact valve complex offers the only available operative alternative.

When selecting patients for this operation, it is important to establish that the reflux is "axial" and does not involve parallel channels. In these instances, interposition of a single competent valve can alleviate symptoms. Otherwise, valve reconstruction at multiple levels is necessary to prevent retrograde flow through parallel incompetent venous segments. The function of cryopreserved valved segments may allow the latter approach to be pursued.

*Venous Valve Transposition*

## OPERATIVE PROCEDURE

Venous valve transposition can be offered to carefully selected patients with severe venous valvular incompetence and incapacitating symptoms. Preoperative studies include ascending and descending venography. Duplex ultrasonography can be used to identify an axillary venous segment of appropriate size that contains a competent valve segment. The basilic vein becomes the axillary vein as it crosses the border of the teres major muscle, and it provides an acceptable donor source when large.

With the patient under general anesthesia, the upper arm and affected leg are sterilely prepared and draped. A longitudinal incision is made over the donor axillary or basilic venous segment (Fig. 248). A large tributary commonly joins the vein at the site of the venous valve, and this branch must be carefully ligated and divided without disturbing the valve or its supporting structure. The donor segment is removed, leaving an ample length of vein proximal and distal to the valve that is sufficient to allow beveling and anastomosis without damage to the valve.

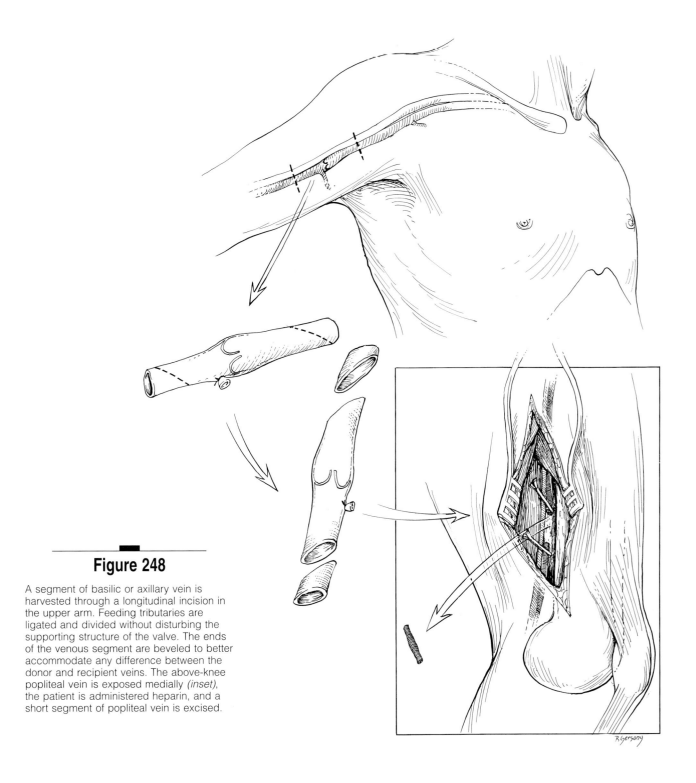

## Figure 248

A segment of basilic or axillary vein is
harvested through a longitudinal incision in
the upper arm. Feeding tributaries are
ligated and divided without disturbing the
supporting structure of the valve. The ends
of the venous segment are beveled to better
accommodate any difference between the
donor and recipient veins. The above-knee
popliteal vein is exposed medially *(inset)*,
the patient is administered heparin, and a
short segment of popliteal vein is excised.

R. Gersony

### Venous Valve Transposition

The site of valve insertion is chosen on the basis of the preoperative imaging studies. We have found the above-knee popliteal vein to be the most appropriate location for a single valve transposition because large, parallel venous channels are uncommon at this level. This segment is exposed through an approach identical to that used for exposure of the suprageniculai popliteal artery. The patient is administered heparin, and a short length of vein is excised, remembering that the ends will retract and increase the distance to be bridged by the interposed axillary venous segment. Measurement of the lengths of these venous segments before division helps avoid tension or redundancy.

A length of externally supported prosthetic conduit slightly larger than the venous diameter is used to prevent dilatation of the interposed valve segment and possible recurrence of venous reflux. The segment is threaded over the popliteal vein before beginning the anastomoses (Fig. 249). The donor segment is then interposed, completing each beveled end-to-end anastomosis with fine polypropylene suture. "Purse-stringing" of the anastomotic suture line must be avoided to prevent narrowing. The prosthetic sleeve is then advanced over the donor segment, and the wounds are closed.

Protamine sulfate is not used, and postoperative heparinization is continued until the patient is adequately anticoagulated with warfarin. External pneumatic compression applied distal to the transposition site is a useful adjunctive measure until the patient is ambulatory. An elastic wrap over the arm wound discourages hematoma formation.

## Figure 249

*A,* A sleeve of externally supported PTFE conduit is threaded over the recipient vein. *B,* The donor segment is interposed, completing each anastomosis with fine polypropylene suture. Care must be exercised to avoid narrowing of the vessel during construction of the anastomoses. The anastomotic suture must not catch the valve leaflet or alter its supporting structure. *C,* The PTFE sleeve is advanced over the donor segment to prevent later dilatation with recurrent venous reflux.

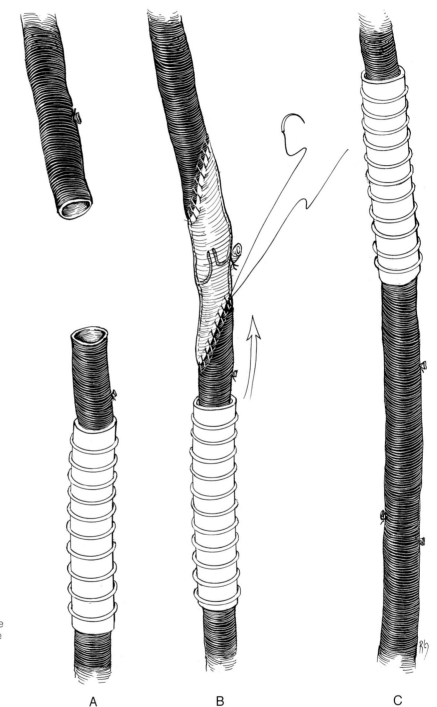

A  B  C

# CHAPTER 40

# Iliac Venous Thrombectomy

Acute iliofemoral venous thrombosis is associated with a higher incidence of complications than deep venous thromboses at other levels, including pulmonary embolism and post-thrombotic sequelae. The propensity for late post-thrombotic complications reflects the lower recanalization rates in the iliofemoral segment, with dilation of distal valves below the obstruction and secondary incompetence of otherwise uninvolved segments. Early removal of thrombus can result in immediate and long-term clinical improvement.

An important consideration in treating iliofemoral venous thrombosis is the likelihood of an underlying anatomic lesion, frequently a narrowing in the form of a venous web or synechia developing where the left iliac vein crosses beneath the right common iliac artery. Failure to address such underlying venous pathology often results in rethrombosis.

There are two appropriate methods for re-establishing flow through the occluded iliofemoral venous segment: thrombolysis and thrombectomy. Venous thrombolysis is best accomplished through catheter-directed techniques. Earlier methods employed systemic infusions of a thrombolytic agent, but catheter access from the contralateral femoral vein, a jugular vein, or the ipsilateral popliteal vein (the preferred route of access) allow high-dose local urokinase infusion to effect prompt and more complete lysis.

Venous thrombectomy, although less likely to remove thrombus lodged in small peripheral venous tributaries, provides a rapid method of clearing the main segments. The operative results can be dramatic, with almost instantaneous resolution of edema, discoloration, and pain. When applied soon after thrombosis, it can achieve long-term patency and preservation of valve function.

## OPERATIVE PROCEDURE

Regardless of the choice of intervention, the patient is administered heparin as soon as the diagnosis of iliofemoral venous thrombosis is made. With the patient under general endotracheal anesthesia with positive pressure ventilation, the groin is sterilely prepared and draped.

Femoral venous exposure is obtained on the affected side, controlling the common femoral, superficial femoral, profunda, and saphenous segments (Fig. 250). A transverse femoral venotomy is made just above the profunda inflow. A venous thrombectomy catheter of appropriate size is introduced and advanced into the inferior vena cava. The catheter is withdrawn, extracting the thrombus and achieving brisk venous backflow.

Adequacy of the thrombectomy and the absence of residual anatomic lesions should be confirmed by contrast venography. Any underlying venous lesions should be addressed immediately to prevent early rethrombosis. Operative patch angioplasty, division, and reanastomosis of the right iliac artery to translocate the artery beneath the iliac vein or (most commonly) endoluminal stenting is usually necessary.

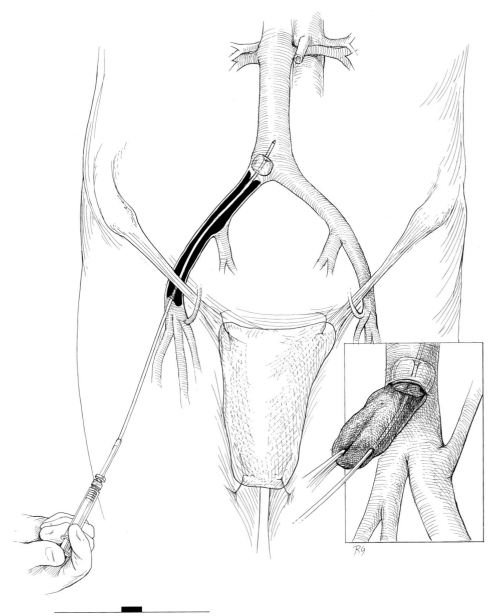

## Figure 250

Iliac venous thrombectomy is performed through a common femoral venotomy by passing a venous thrombectomy balloon catheter to extrude the thrombus.

## Iliac Venous Thrombectomy

Balloon catheter thrombectomy is usually not feasible below the femoral venotomy because of competent venous valves that obstruct the progress of the catheter. Attempts to do so will damage the very valves whose function needs to be preserved. In early cases, however, application of an Esmarch bandage and massage results in prompt extrusion of the offending thrombus from the open venotomy.

Except in very early cases, it is wise to construct a temporary arteriovenous fistula at the conclusion of an iliac venous thrombectomy. This has proved efficacious in randomized trials. A large tributary of the saphenous vein may provide a suitable means of temporarily increasing flow across the thrombectomized iliac vein (Fig. 251), but if unavailable, the greater saphenous vein itself can be employed. In either case, an end-to-side anastomosis is constructed between the vein and the common femoral artery.

The fistula is left open for 2 to 4 weeks, until venous re-endothelialization has occurred. At this point, the fistula is occluded, preferably by endovascular means. Contrast injection at this time can confirm patency of the thrombectomized segment. Alternatively, a polypropylene suture doubly looped around the fistula, brought out to the skin, and tied over a button can serve as an easy means of later fistula ligation.

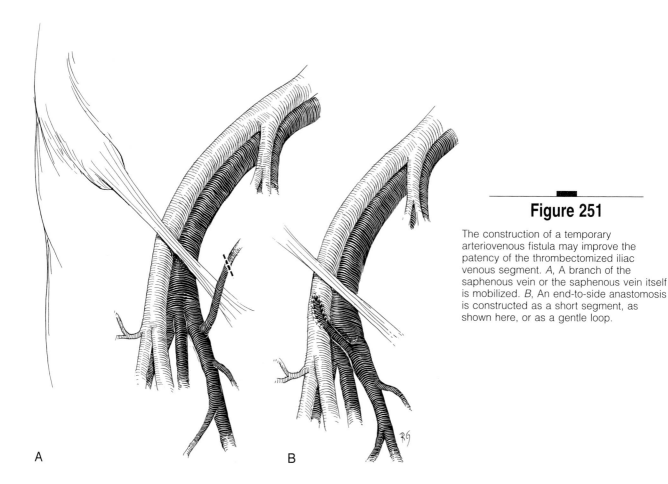

A          B

### Figure 251

The construction of a temporary arteriovenous fistula may improve the patency of the thrombectomized iliac venous segment. *A,* A branch of the saphenous vein or the saphenous vein itself is mobilized. *B,* An end-to-side anastomosis is constructed as a short segment, as shown here, or as a gentle loop.

# CHAPTER 41

# Iliac Venous Bypass

Patients with obstruction of the iliac vein present initially with massive leg edema, cyanosis, and pain. These individuals may eventually become relatively asymptomatic if adequate collateral channels develop, limiting venous hypertension. If the peripheral venous valves remain competent, the patient may avoid the post-thrombotic syndrome. Occasionally, however, poorly collateralized iliac vein occlusion produces persistent, incapacitating leg edema and venous claudication. In these cases, venous bypass may be associated with prompt and lasting relief of symptoms. These are patients in whom the opportunities for early thrombus removal were missed.

Candidates for venous bypass procedures should undergo venography to accurately define the anatomy of the femoral and iliac venous segments. Pressure measurements should be obtained at this time. Venous bypass grafts are unlikely to be needed or remain patent in the absence of a significant resting pressure gradient (e.g., 10 mm Hg) between the ipsilateral femoral vein and the inferior vena cava. The absence of a significant gradient suggests that the pathophysiology may be more related to venous valvular incompetence than outflow obstruction. Ambulatory venous pressure recordings or plethysmography can aid in making this determination.

Operative results are poor when a femoral vein has been recanalized, because it makes a poor anastomotic inflow site. The best long-term outcome is obtained when the infrainguinal venous system is relatively normal. In this regard, established stasis changes in the lower leg also predict a poor response to venous bypass, because they indicate the coexistence of venous valvular dysfunction. Surgical relief of outflow obstruction alone cannot alter the outlook for such patients.

Several operative options are available for treating symptomatic iliac venous occlusion. The saphenous vein crossover graft represents a logical and theoretically pleasing method of relieving outflow obstruction. The saphenous vein, however, may not be large enough to provide a sufficient route of outflow. We have employed prosthetic bypass grafts as an alternative, using externally supported (ringed) ePTFE conduits to bridge the gap between a near-normal femoral system and the inferior vena cava. If the obstruction is hemodynamically significant, with pressure gradients exhibited at rest, such conduits enjoy satisfactory long-term patency.

*Iliac Venous Bypass*

## OPERATIVE PROCEDURE

The patient is positioned on the operating table with a bolster beneath the right flank (Fig. 252). With the patient under regional or general anesthesia, the common femoral vein is exposed on the affected side (Fig. 253). A right flank incision is used to gain access to the retroperitoneal space, and the ureter and peritoneal contents are retracted medially. A mechanical retractor is of great assistance in obtaining adequate exposure of the inferior vena cava. A 10- to 12-mm, ringed ePTFE graft is tunneled between the groin incision and the right retroperitoneum. Although the tunnel is easily developed from the right groin, creating a tunnel from the left groin can be treacherous. The surgeon should carefully follow the route of the left iliac artery, digitally developing the tunnel from the retroperitoneum and groin.

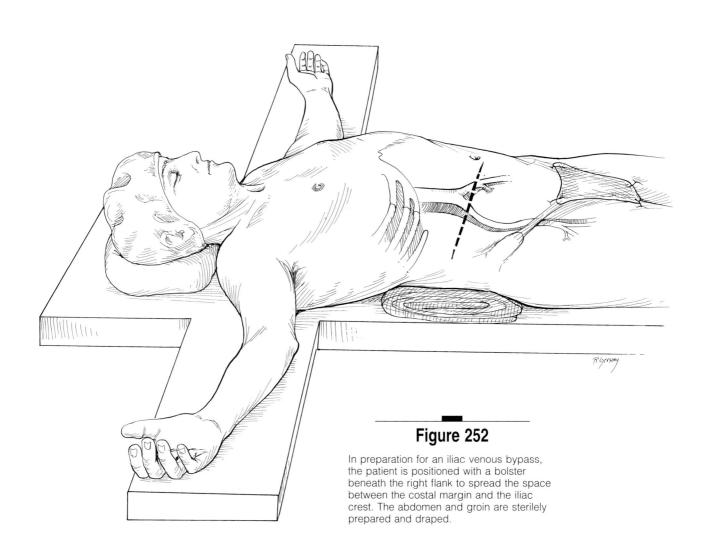

### Figure 252

In preparation for an iliac venous bypass, the patient is positioned with a bolster beneath the right flank to spread the space between the costal margin and the iliac crest. The abdomen and groin are sterilely prepared and draped.

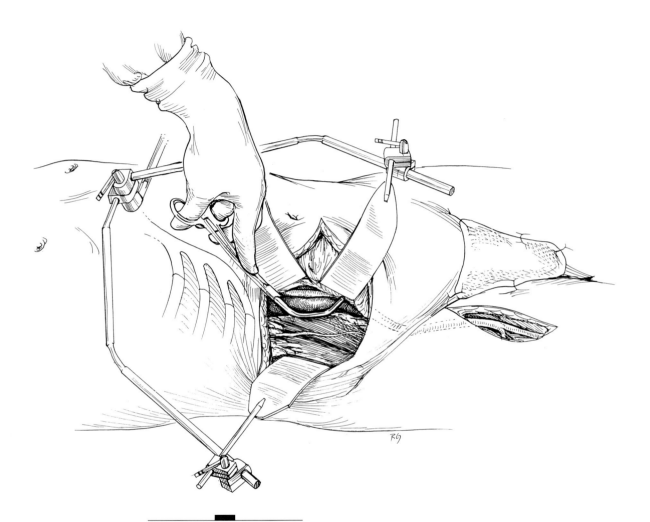

**Figure 253**

Using a mechanical retractor, the peritoneal sac is retracted medially, along with the right ureter. The vena cava is exposed over its anterior and lateral aspects without gaining individual control of the lumbar veins. The common femoral vein is exposed in the affected extremity, and an 8- or 10-mm ringed ePTFE graft is tunneled retroperitoneally.

## Iliac Venous Bypass

The patient is administered heparin, and the inferior vena cava is clamped. A clamp of the Satinsky variety provides effective control, obviating the need to individually control each lumbar vein (Fig. 254). The caval anastomosis is constructed with 5-0 or 6-0 Gore-Tex suture. The femoral anastomosis is performed with 7-0 Gore-Tex suture, using a side-biting clamp to avoid separate control of the profunda femoris vein and numerous dilated collateral tributaries (Fig. 255). Occasionally, the femoral vein is more diseased than suspected on the basis of the preoperative venogram. Synechiae can be divided and an endophlebectomy performed, but the long-term prospects are poorer for this subset of patients.

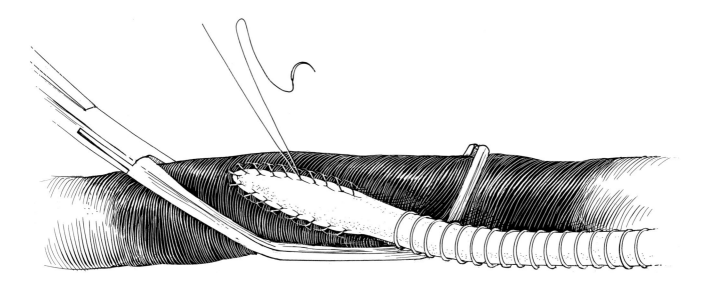

**Figure 254**

The caval anastomosis is completed with
5-0 or 6-0 Gore-Tex suture.

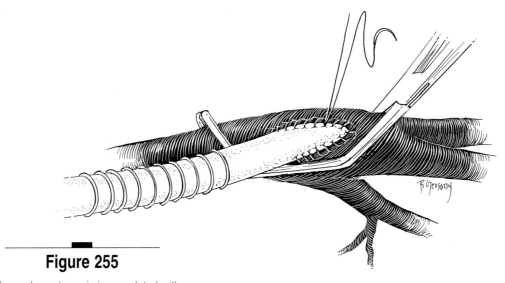

**Figure 255**

The femoral anastomosis is completed with
7-0 Gore-Tex suture.

## Iliac Venous Bypass

The clamps are released after completion of the anastomoses (Fig. 256), and pressures within the femoral vein and vena cava are again measured. No pressure gradient should be detected when the technical result is adequate. A temporary arteriovenous fistula may be constructed to improve patency (see Chapter 40). Anticoagulation may or may not be reversed with protamine sulfate, depending on hemostasis within the retroperitoneum. The wounds are closed, and low-dose heparin therapy is instituted, increasing to a therapeutic dose within 24 to 48 hours postoperatively. Long-term oral anticoagulation is continued as long as the graft remains patent.

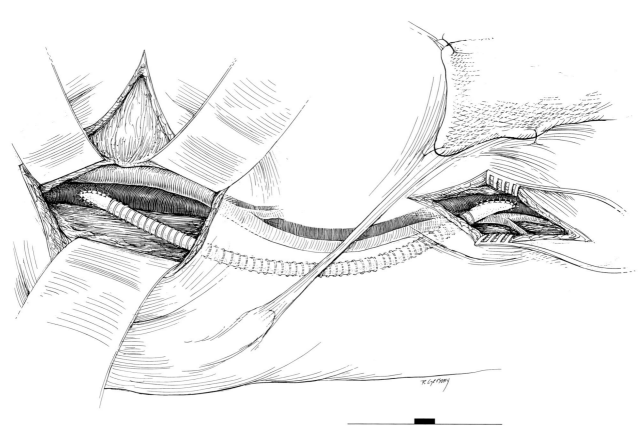

**Figure 256**

The graft lies in its retroperitoneal tunnel.

# INDEX

**281**

ISBN 0-7216-6994-8

90038